The Promise

A Walk of Faith
along the IVF Journey

TODD A. REHNQUIST

Halo
PUBLISHING
INTERNATIONAL

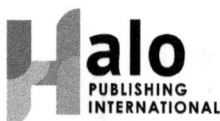

Halo
PUBLISHING
INTERNATIONAL

Halo Publishing International
8000 W Interstate 10, #600
San Antonio, Texas 78230

First Edition, September 2022
Printed in the United States of America
ISBN 978-1-63765-284-8
Library of Congress Control Number: 2022913387

Halo Publishing International is a self-publishing company that publishes adult fiction and non-fiction, children's literature, self-help, spiritual, and faith-based books. We continually strive to help authors reach their publishing goals and provide many different services that help them do so. We do not publish books that are deemed to be politically, religiously, or socially disrespectful, or books that are sexually provocative, including erotica. Halo reserves the right to refuse publication of any manuscript if it is deemed not to be in line with our principles. Do you have a book idea you would like us to consider publishing? Please visit www.halopublishing.com for more information.

I dedicate this writing to my wife, Nataliya.
To those little ones she brought forth, Abigail and Ella.
To God's promise, His continued faithfulness,
and all He led us through.

Contents

Chapter 1 Cuppa Joe?   11

Chapter 2 Nataliya's Treasure Chest   14

Chapter 3 Finding Peace in Her Heart   17

Chapter 4 The Revelation of God's Promise   21

Chapter 5 How Do I Receive This News?   24

Chapter 6 What Is a Promise?   30

Chapter 7 In Real Time–August   35

Chapter 8 The Goal Still Attainable?   45

Chapter 9 Believing God in the Midst of Trauma   48

Chapter 10 A Change of Plans   51

Chapter 11 Ready   56

Chapter 12 Launch   58

Chapter 13 Proven   60

Chapter 14 On the Road Again   62

Chapter 15 One More Door   64

Chapter 16 Praying   67

Chapter 17 Praying More!   69

Chapter 18 Enough!   73

Chapter 19 'A More Real Time'   76

Chapter 20 One Week Later   77

Chapter 21 Onward   82

Chapter 22 To Move One Forward   84

Chapter 23 On the Path Again   85

Chapter 24 A Very Special Easter Egg   89

Chapter 25 Five Months Along   92

Chapter 26 I Asked Them to Pray   94

Chapter 27 A Quiverful–Two Years Later   96

Chapter 28 Taken by Faith   112

Chapter 29 Second Trimester   114

Chapter 30 Joy   115

Chapter 31 A Journey Filled with Every Emotion   118

Chapter 32 The Third *T*   120

Chapter 33 One Week or Less   121

Chapter 34 Arrived   123

Chapter 35 A Message of Hope   124

Chapter 1

Cuppa Joe?

Our friends are more than just occasional fun company. The really good ones are a source of comfort and guidance. I am blessed to have several good friends, as I hope you have, yet when my wife and I went through one of our most challenging times, I did not turn to any of them for advice. After all, none of them had been through the in vitro fertilization (IVF) path we were in the midst of traveling.

Yes, there are a few who would have willingly listened attentively to our plight. Once we began to share some of the details of the path that brought our daughter to us, there were those who seemed hurt and surprised that we had not included them from the beginning. Their reactions validated our choice. We could only imagine the extra pressure involved if we had to answer well-meaning questions from several people on the days when failure and sadness overtook us. It would have only magnified the emotional trauma we underwent.

God is always there for me. As we read in Psalm 23:4, "Even when the way goes through Death Valley, I'm not afraid when you walk at my side. Your trusty shepherd's crook makes me feel secure." And He certainly accompanied us during this journey of faith. Yet there are times we all crave human understanding in companionship. If only I'd had a friend, brother, mentor who could have sat down with me to share a cup of coffee. Someone who'd been there before. Someone who could prepare me for what was to come and console me for all that passed.

Now that I have come out on the other side of the promise of new life, I want to be the friend I did not have. I want to sit with you and share my story so that you may have a glimpse into what may await you on the IVF journey, so that you may have a friend who understands what you are about to face—a friend who says, "You are not alone. You can do this. Have faith."

So pour a cup of coffee and travel through the pages of this book, and I will share our journey with you.

I applaud those of you who endure life's most difficult struggles and are willing to write about and share them. Revisiting the events and details of life-changing moments in order to record them for others can make us live them afresh. Make us feel the pain and the joy all over again. So personal, and yet a balm to the writer's soul, is to write of trauma and joy, those things that exist in the moments of life's greatest difficulties and triumphs. What is written here, this story, is real.

As we tread the path of life's journey, it is important to keep trusting God and His promises. We must continue standing together, as my wife and I did, pressing through, persevering in the beliefs that life would come forth and that through the trials awaiting us, we would be rewarded.

I ask him to strengthen you by his Spirit—not a brute strength but a glorious inner strength—that Christ will live in you as you open the door and invite him in. And I ask him that with both feet planted firmly on love you'll be able to take in with all Christians the extravagant dimensions of Christ's love. Reach out and experience the breadth! Test its length! Plumb the depths! Rise to the heights! (Ephesians 3:16–18)

My wife, Nataliya, brought her vision to me, and guided by my faith in God, I said yes in response to the process that would bring us two darling, lovely, beautiful little girls—the promises of God fulfilled.

Chapter 2

Nataliya's Treasure Chest

It would be sensitive to describe Nataliya and me as "older" parents, as is so often the case with couples who embark on the IVF journey. The average age of first-time fathers is thirty-one, while the average age of first-time mothers is twenty-seven.[1] Suffice it to say, we are both older than those averages. Having another child was not a topic of conversation in our household, and after eight years of marriage, it was an unspoken and accepted fact that it never would be an option up for discussion. I was a father and grandfather from a previous marriage, and thoughts of having another baby were nonexistent, so much so that I had undergone a vasectomy nine years before I met Nataliya.

---

[1] https://www.webmd.com/infertility-and-reproduction/news/20210831/men-over-50-less-likely-have-baby-ivf

In January of 2014, Nataliya attended a five-day school for ministers and lay leaders at the Ministries of Pastoral Care (MPC) in Wheaton, Illinois. Attendees go there to "learn about and experience how we are healed through Christ's work on the Cross and the Holy Spirit's real presence with and within us."[2]

During her time there, Nataliya performed an exercise in which everyone was asked to participate.

"Picture in your mind," the leader said, "you're out in the ocean, on a boat, getting ready to dive over the edge. Now, hold your breath as you're diving downward to the bottom. As you get closer to the bottom, a treasure chest becomes visible, one the Lord Jesus placed there for you. The treasure within is something that you have a deep longing for, but have forgotten about. The pressures of life on Earth have erased your heart's true desires. Life has hidden your hopes, and the treasure chest you will see resting on the bottom is holding that desire, the one stored deep in your soul."

As the exercise unfolded, Nataliya visualized herself kicking her feet, diving deeper, until she arrived at the bottom of the ocean. She grasped the lid of the box, but it would not open. It wouldn't even budge the tiniest amount as she slogged it from side to side. Just as she felt she was completely running out of air, the Lord gently spoke to her, "Take the chest to the top where the boat is."

In her mind, she replied, "It is too heavy; I can't lift it." But, using the last of her air, Nataliya tried one more time, and the chest broke free from the barnacles that ensnared it; she couldn't

---

[2] https://ministriesofpastoralcare.com/schools/

believe how light it was. She quickly swam back to the surface, hoisted the chest onto the deck of the boat, and climbed in after it.

Nataliya crouched down and lifted the lid. Inside was a beautiful, multicolored Easter egg with a seam around it so it could be easily opened, similar to the plastic eggs hidden for children's Easter-egg hunts.

She gently opened the egg, and there was a baby inside. She handed the baby to Jesus, who was suddenly standing next to her.

He blessed the child. It was then that she heard the voice of God. "Who made the choice when you said you were done having children? Was that Me—God—or you who made that choice without Me?"

Chapter 3

Finding Peace in Her Heart

Nataliya did not rush home to tell me of her vision. For six months, she held this revelation close to her heart, sharing it with only one other person. She sought the guidance of our long-term friend and professional counselor, Barbra. Barbra had counseled us during the early years of our marriage and continues to be a supportive friend to both of us. Barbra held Nataliya's secret.

Nataliya wasn't sure if she should share her vision with me. And if she did, how would she choose the words to tell me? A child was not on our radar. How would I receive the news?

It may not be lost on you, as it certainly wasn't on me later, that my Nataliya was facing the same dilemma as Mary did in Luke 1:30–38.

But the angel assured her, "Mary, you have nothing to fear. God has a surprise for you. You will become pregnant and give birth to a son and call his name Jesus. He will be great, be called Son of the Highest. The Lord God will give him the throne of his father David; He will rule Jacob's house forever—no end, ever, to his kingdom."

Mary said to the angel, "But how? I've never slept with a man."

The angel answered, "The Holy Spirit will come upon you, the power of the Highest hover over you; Therefore, the child you bring to birth will be called Holy, Son of God. And did you know that your cousin Elizabeth conceived a son, old as she is? Everyone called her barren, and here she is six months pregnant! Nothing, you see, is impossible with God."

And Mary said, "Yes, I see it all now. I'm the Lord's maid, ready to serve. Let it be with me just as you say."

Then the angel left her.

The similarities are remarkable between Mary and Nataliya. Both are given a vision and a promise from God that a child will be coming forth. Pregnancy is an impossibility for both—Mary as a virgin and Nataliya with a husband who has had a vasectomy. Mary must find a way to tell Joseph, with whom she hasn't lain, and Nataliya must find a way to tell me, her husband who has already made his mind up about the issue. How does one do that and overcome the fear of being rejected?

Barbra's advice to Nataliya was, "You need to have peace in your heart first; Todd can say no to this revelation, and everyone will still be okay afterwards."

The larger question at hand: Would Nataliya be okay afterwards if Todd's answer is no? Could she really find the peace that she needed?

Nataliya had discovered within herself the deeper reasons for not pursuing her desire to have more children. As if hermetically sealed away, hidden from all human purpose or attachment to a cause, even her own deepest desire of having more children was hidden from herself.

It took six months of prayer and waiting, and in that time, Nataliya made another visit to Wheaton and the Ministries of Pastoral Care. Once again, she heard the voice of God speaking to her heart, His promise emphasized—the promise of a child.

I see more clearly now the impact of what happened to her in a previous relationship. Likely something that has happened to many other women too. Having had a child in a prior marriage and having suffered the pain and anguish of a difficult divorce had hardened Nataliya's heart against future progeny. The desire for another child and a vow "not to" were hidden, the profundity of which, no man, only God knows. Yes, it would take God himself to uncover this hidden desire buried deep in her heart. To show her the true reason for its being sealed away. A vow she made to herself to never again procreate. Truth is, being hurt by another had caused the schism, separating her from her true wish and need, hiding them away even from herself.

This showed me even more that, to have an intellectual understanding that God's promises are not to be taken lightly, nor are they to be rejected, ignored, or disbelieved, is one thing. But to have the faith to believe in God's promises asks so much more of us. The unearthing that only He could accomplish through the process of receiving the word brought to hearts at an MPC conference—or in Nataliya's case, believing it and having the faith to have another child with the man she's now married to, me.

No matter how strong one's faith is in God's promises, the IVF journey will test you repeatedly and sometimes savagely. Tears must fall on this blessed and precarious road.

As our journey progressed, I would find comfort in Genesis 17:16–17.

> *"I'll bless her—yes! I'll give you a son by her! Oh, how I'll bless her! Nations will come from her; kings of nations will come from her."*
>
> *Abraham fell flat on his face. And then he laughed, thinking, "Can a hundred-year-old man father a son? And can Sarah, at ninety years, have a baby?"*

With Abraham and Sarah's story in mind, the possibility seemed more real; after all, I was certainly less than a hundred years old.

Chapter 4

The Revelation of God's Promise

Unlike biblical revelations, we weren't on a mountaintop, and there were no burning bushes or blaring trumpets. On an otherwise average Thursday night, Nataliya was ready to tell me of her revelation and the promise God had delivered to her.

How does one even begin to share a promise of this nature? Simply by faith, I guess, the variable that changes lives forever. The only variable that continues to do so—faith. So when Nataliya gathered the words—or, more accurately, the song sang over her and illustrated how to compose those words—to tell me what God had shown her, His promise, the words deep within her heart made entry into the world. She shared the assurance she received in her January 2014 encounter with the Lord.

We were in the living room when Nataliya began with, "Come over here, and sit down. I want to talk to you, share with you about some stuff, you know? I've met with Barbra about this, and there's something I want to talk to you about."

As she began to speak, my frightened husband's mind could tell we were launching into a very serious conversation. My first thought was, *She is trying to tell me that she is leaving me.*

But, instead, Nataliya reminded me of her trip to the Ministries of Pastoral Care six months prior. I managed to focus on her words and not my fears as she told the rest of the story.

She retold the visualization of diving to the bottom of the sea so vividly I too could see it in my mind's eye. When Nataliya returned to the boat, I was standing there with her, dripping salt water onto the deck.

The impact of what she was relating to me didn't register until she said, "Todd, this is God telling us that we are to have a child."

Emotionally, we were off the charts. Nataliya had six months to sit with this news of God's promise. I was trying to absorb it all within minutes.

At first, I was distracted by my relief that she wasn't leaving me. You may be thinking there was a scene. You may be thinking I stormed off and had to be alone. You may be thinking I asked her for some time to think about such a big decision, an event that would make a huge impact on our lives. But that is not how it unfolded.

My thought was, *How can I not say yes?* I said to Nataliya, "You want this. Obviously, the Lord has found this in your heart somewhere, something that's been there, buried underneath a lot of other stuff, life."

She's my spouse, and I love her, and I want what she wants. Whenever she has asked me about anything in our lives, it has added to our relationship, benefited us, and not hurt us.

Whether it was planning a weekend getaway at the Ritz to unwind when I had been working too hard, or getting an outside office for my business after having worked from home for the past twenty years, we had always come out better when we heeded her suggestions. This time, her request just happened to be a child.

Within forty-five minutes, I was looking around the house, which had only one bedroom on the main floor, and saying, "We're going to need a different house."

Chapter 5

How Do I Receive This News?

For me, analogously, the promise to Sarah and the one seemingly staring me down at that time were the same. My first step would be to believe what God had promised Nataliya. Did I question that she had this experience? Not in that moment, and at no point ever, did it cross my mind to doubt her.

We have a solid eight-year marriage in which we both stand with trust and faith—a marriage that has been tested, tried, and proven. It has withstood the pressure of life's daily demands—the demands that impact our very souls, our minds, emotions, and wills. All the while, God watches over this crucible (our lives in the tangible world). Facing those difficulties and happenstances together and making the necessary sacrifices that they demand allows room for a better, stronger life.

Removing the slag, I call it. That stony waste material separated during the smelting or refining of ore, or in this life, it's better known as our will versus His.

God scrapes off that old slag that comes to the top, purifying us more and more. Our marriages, in so many ways, become better when yielding to the process.

I don't know about you, but *my wife—the same as precious metals being put through the fire, becoming more pliable and valuable—has made my life better by speaking the truth of God into me, into our marriage.*

Most men, I believe, if truthful, would admit their lives have become better because of what their wives have spoken into them. In my marriage—learning to live together, growing in trust, believing in one another more and more as the years pass by—I am the benefactor of having a wife like this.

But this was about more than just my belief in something that happened to Nataliya. *By hearing her revelation, I have now been invited to partake in its unfoldment. I have the choice to accept and partake. I also have the choice to decline, thereby denying Nataliya...and God as well? After all, God didn't speak to me about this.*

Did Joseph wonder the same thing? Joseph was presented with the fait accompli, whereas I have free will to bring forth a child. Which is more difficult? To accept a fate that has been decreed by God, or have the free will to turn it down? Would my denial be a denial of my faith? My marriage? My promise to both my wife and to God?

Forsaking all others was a promise I made to my wife on the day of our wedding. Am I not myself considered an "other"? Joseph forsook himself for the sake of his wife, Mary. He could have stoned her to death and been applauded for doing so according to the culture of the time. Before truly understanding he had a choice, he chose to accept as truth Mary's telling of the event that caused her to become pregnant, even though he was troubled about it—talk about faith! I too had a choice, but only one choice, just like Joseph. Only one that would bring us closer.

Forsaking myself for my wife—her ideas, her thoughts, and her heart have always worked out better for us. Every time I have chosen "not me" in most of the larger issues we've faced together, it has worked out better for us and our family, and better for me personally. I know my wife. She is a woman of faith. I applaud her for having the courage to speak out of that faith about something that would change our lives, always for the better.

Matthew 1:18–24 shows us that Joseph indeed had doubts.

> *The birth of Jesus took place like this. His mother, Mary, was engaged to be married to Joseph. Before they came to the marriage bed, Joseph discovered she was pregnant. (It was by the Holy Spirit, but he didn't know that.) Joseph, chagrined but noble, determined to take care of things quietly so Mary would not be disgraced. While he was trying to figure a way out, he had a dream.*

> *God's angel spoke in the dream: "Joseph, son of David, don't hesitate to get married. Mary's pregnancy is Spirit-conceived. God's Holy Spirit has made her pregnant. She will bring a son to birth, and when she does, you, Joseph, will name him Jesus—God saves—because he will save his people from their sins."*

> *This would bring the prophet's embryonic sermon to full term: Watch for this—a virgin will get pregnant and bear a son. They will name him Emmanuel. (Hebrew for "God is with us.")*

Then Joseph woke up. He did exactly what God's angel commanded in the dream. He married Mary.

What would be next for us if I were to receive the promise granted to Nataliya? Many have been exposed to such grandeur, not knowing that it was the voice of God speaking to their most inward self, and yet a family's increase came through the power of that word placed gently within them.

This would take a gargantuan leap of faith for me, but only when I received what God made known to Nataliya would it be granted. The promise of increase, a child to be added to our family—an incredible thought. Later, I too would receive a vision about the changing dynamics of our family.

What a whirlwind that night was for me. To have enough faith to believe Nataliya's story, the promise the Lord had given her, it took my breath away, leaving a void that needed to be filled.

Hearing the story was a pivotal moment. Through my hearing, the circuit was made complete—followed by faith—then believing. For isn't this the way that the Lord works—faith, believing, and then result?

The genesis of thought was conceived now in our household. As if this news weren't enough for one to grapple with, the timing was huge. Is there ever a good time for the explosion of thought that might change one's life? A child? Most certainly, no small change. It was the greatest of things in our lives at that time. A promise spoken by God, going into the heart of another human being that day. I suspect it had the same effect as Mary's acceptance, which is found in the Scriptures—God's promise in Luke 1:38 when Mary said to the angel, "Let it be unto me according to your word." And that of my wife, God's promise to her, and now to me. Let it be unto me, her husband, to have faith and believe.

My wife believed and received. And as Mary carried this great weight in her heart to share with Joseph, telling her husband the promise from God, my wife's turn came, just as Mary's did. Sharing, laying it at my feet, similar as Mary's was laid at Joseph's feet. The similarity is astonishing. For she and I were now yoked together in a new way because I had believed. It changed everything in the makeup of our family.

Nataliya had carried the promise, her vision, for months, and on that evening it became her revelation to me. And now, I too would shepherd this promise.

A heavy weight is lightened for her, for now we both carry the poundage together. The load was meant to be lighter with two becoming one in the promise of God. A threefold chord becomes as it should, one stronger, one resolute, one now struck, resonating a joyous harmony.

But to carry more was upon the horizon for us, for we had just refinanced our home prior to this news—the promise now harmonizing within our hearts. Moving again wasn't even on the radar, and yet those course corrections were beginning for us. Immediately, our minds turned toward making room for the addition to our family. We knew we wanted a house with two bedrooms on the main floor, so we weren't navigating the stairs day and night.

Prior to the promise, a common goal we shared was one that many look forward to one day—paying off our mortgage. For us, that was a goal that could be reached in the next several years. The view suddenly changed for us.

The promise had not only changed our goals, it changed the way we see. It changed the things we'd placed value on.

We both agreed that a move was necessary for us to have another child. So we decided to sell our home, even though we refinanced only months earlier. Moving was something we never thought we'd do, at least anytime soon. The promise was now already making changes. It began to shape most of what we did and saw, requiring a change in direction to fulfill it.

We would believe God and step to whatever direction He would lead—sometimes joyfully, sometimes not.

We were on the same page moving forward. We agreed rapidly to a new home and a new child. We had no idea what challenges awaited us.

Chapter 6

What Is a Promise?

I've spoken many times already about the promise that was given to Nataliya and me—God's promise. Over the course of the days and years that have followed Nataliya's revelation, I have examined the concept of "promise" extensively. This scrutiny begins with questions: What is a promise? When do you know a promise is real? How can you trust one when it is made? Does it have more than one meaning? Does it mean something different for each person?

"Promise" is one of those words that is both a noun and a verb. One may issue a promise, as if it were a gift, a bunch of flowers, or box of candy. One may extract a promise, as if holding someone to a contract—"Do you promise to be here by eight o'clock?"

Of course, there is the act of giving the promise. So a promise is an ongoing thing if one truly commits to it. It requires faith and allegiance, and in some cases tenacity, to follow a promise through to completion.

Think of the promise ring. It is a gift sometimes exchanged between young couples of high school or college age. It symbolizes their promise to stay together and to one day replace the promise ring with an engagement ring.

Engagement, too, is a promise. A promise to exclude all others and to marry at a future date.

Marriage is a promise of devotion. Marriage is entered into in the eyes of God and includes God in the relationship. Two become one in God.

You're probably asking your own questions right now—such as, "Why is the author assuming my familiarity with this theorem—of a promise made, and then having that promise broken?" The answer is, I'm writing to people who live their lives on the same planet I do. Those who've been exposed as I've been. Just to live is to have experienced a broken promise; it is a certainty. It is necessary and relevant to explore the importance of defining this theorem before continuing with our story.

In my life, probably yours too, a broken promise is not only likely to occur, but most probable. For many, it already has, and more than once. So the theorem proven, living side by side with other human beings, day in and day out, people simply miss the mark at times with promises—those made and those kept. We even break promises that we make to ourselves.

This just happens. We've all experienced, more than once most of us, people breaking their commitments. Causing us not to trust, in the end, those who are now mature adults. We are left skeptical about committing with confidence. Commitment becomes a most hated thing when the infringing deceit transgresses our selfhood, which is now fully grown. It sets us up to never trust again, and we begin creating boundaries - allowing others we don't fully trust to make promises to us - to avoid the pain associated with this - throughout our lives to protect ourselves.

And yet, those boundaries are breached. Why are we still subject? We are subject, meaning "exposed" because we live alongside all human beings collectively on planet Earth. We fight to overcome the loss of trust we once had in others, ourselves, even God, oftentimes taking a lifetime to mend—some of us never do. Yet until this broken trust is mended, it leaves one not only guarded, but leading a more narrow life. With an opaque belief of being alive, when in reality they are just existing. How do we move past the brutality of betrayal? We begin questioning the motives of those around us, causing ourselves anxiety. We come to expect more betrayal.

When we hear others say, "I promise," regarding that which really matters most to us, it ushers in a knee-jerk reaction and the self-protection engine light flashing on the dash of one's soul—"Yield! Remember last time!" And it remains lit until the apology comes. Yes, we wait for the balm of healing to be applied, wait for it to make its way inward, downward, healing a severed trust, a broken heart. We wait for that healing, hoping it will come, relatives and friendships restored.

Based on my experience, until this balm is received, the hope will continue to languish in those who believed when another said, "I promise," only to have that word broken.

Belief

The product of God's promise, a child, waits for belief, and we, Nataliya and I, must act for it to become true. It comes no other way. Belief and action are the foundational byproducts of faith.

To receive the promise, we needed to overcome doubt. We needed to believe. It is sometimes easier to forgive than to forget the past. It is difficult to truly believe we've been forgiven when we feel deep down that, not just others, but God has failed us, has broken His promise. But that is a misconception held by those still learning to know His name, His word, and His ways—all of which are unbreakable.

We had to continually remind ourselves that God is utterly faithful to His promises, even if humans are not. And in this process of recollection, His ways were revealed to us with new dynamics and greater importance—the astonishing promise of a child.

Questions

We questioned daily, incessantly, throughout the process, as will you. *Is this meant to be? When will it happen? Why not us? Why not this time?* And through it all, deep inside, our answer was always vague, but continued our pursuit because of Who made the promise. We find ourselves healed now, having believed through the trauma and difficulty of true life being played out. Healing can come through one's continued struggle to believe, and even be liberating while we wait for outcomes staying on this heading.

A joy-filled life was delivered to us, and we were healed in more ways than we knew, simply because of our steadfast belief in God. This is true and the foundation of not just our story, but many couples' stories. Couples who long for life to come forth, who know they'll have to go through the difficulties of IVF, the madness, and the brokenness that seems to follow such hope.

Going through it, life presented itself tangibly as our adventure began to unfold. We did not know the great difficulties that were waiting for us in the shadows. We discovered the worst and best as Time was dealing the cards and playing its hand.

Why?

So why am I telling you all of this? Why am I exploring a convoluted promise? It's because of the destruction of our ability to trust after a promise is broken and the fallout that breaks down families and friendships. It certainly causes us not to believe in future promises made. Worldly disappointments bring doubt to one who needs God.

Nataliya and I would tinker on the brink of wondering, so much time having gone by, *Is the promise broken, or merely not yet fulfilled?* But the balm was applied more than once, healing us through the promise Jesus made to my wife.

We made it through the storm of doubt, disillusionment, and heartbreak. And whether one believes in God or not, promises will still have there way with all of us.

Chapter 7

In Real Time–August

Everything I'm going to tell you now happened in thirty days. Not one thing more could have fit on our plates without some kind of permanent mental damage to us. And yet, here we are on the other side, and I am grateful for it all.

We put our house on the market and it sold in one week! The buyers' contract gave us thirty days until closing, which meant we had to pack up our four-bedroom house and move out. We needed to find temporary housing before we could even begin our new property search. And for those of you who have been in a similar place, between homes, you know that means putting a large part of your possessions in storage. We were physically and emotionally scattered, but happy.

Once we had a place to lay our heads in a month-by-month apartment rental, we started looking for a site to build our next home and searching for a new school for our eleven-year-old son, Tyler, from Nataliya's previous marriage. Most people would think that putting Tyler in a new school would be fairly easy—just register him in whatever school is designated for the district. But for our son, changing schools was a very big deal. We knew our new home was going to be nearly forty-five minutes away from his current school, and that fact, combined with the news we received from his teacher, seriously impacted our school search.

Tyler's teacher had approached us and said, "Your son needs more help than we can give him." We had no idea what she was talking about, but she went on to say, "Some of the other parents are worried about the way he communicates, because in his attempts to be understood, he touches or grabs people with his hands. It's making the parents nervous."

Many public schools would have let a child with Tyler's issues fall through the cracks. They may have chalked up his actions to a behavior problem, punished him, or isolated him, and never given him another thought. We are grateful the teachers and counselor at Liberty Christian School were knowledgeable enough to recommend we have Tyler tested to identify his learning style. The discovery process opened avenues for us as a family to understand and communicate much better with each other.

To learn more about Tyler and his needs, Nataliya, Tyler, and I went to play therapy. In this type of therapy, one parent and the child go into a playroom, while the therapist and the other parent observe from behind a one-way mirror. The therapist instructed me to sit in a chair in the middle of the toy-filled room and not say anything, and not to start any conversation or ask any questions. The therapist said to wait for Tyler to approach me. She explained that Tyler's mind would be engaged in play, and if I spoke to him, he would have to shut down one side of his brain and shift to the other side to figure out how to answer me. My job was to watch how Tyler played and only respond when he invited me to join him. Tyler's choices with the toys and activities were all about controlling the dolls and figures, a reflection of his communication style in which he is compelled to physically control the exchange.

Tyler was diagnosed as having some of the indications found on the Asperger's syndrome spectrum, with a diagnosis of neurodevelopmental disorder. Its core symptoms are inattention, impulsivity, and hyperactivity, or what is more plainly known as ADHD. This diagnosis guided how we chose his new school. We were fortunate to find a school that welcomed children like Tyler, one where they would not be ignored or bullied, where the staff and structure would be better able to meet his needs. Tyler is now thriving in his new school.

If we had not made the decision to move to an area it turns out is near this school, would Tyler have been given the opportunity to be understood and nurtured in such an excellent academic environment? Perhaps it was all part of His promise.

Packing, moving, house hunting, learning of Tyler's diagnosis, finding a new school—all in 30 days.

With all of that going on, we were making plans to get pregnant. The first step? I would become part of the ten percent of men who decide to have their vasectomy reversed.

After some careful research, we found a urologist in Frisco, Texas, whom we trusted with our story. I mean, how does someone share with just anyone about a promise like that? This was another step leading us forward on the path. Dr. J.B. is regarded as one of the best doctors in this part of the country for vasectomy reversals. At the time, we thought this was the way we were going to proceed. I mean, doesn't this make sense? Not knowing that IVF would be our only chance, and at the same time, not even considering IVF as an option. To what did we say yes? IVF was not even on the radar or an alternative consideration for us. Meaning, you don't know what you don't know. Then, afterwards, you realize you've changed course.

Please, only God could've placed this desire in my heart—to have another child at this stage in my life. I know myself, and I know there is no way that this is my idea.

What were we to do next? We knew a handful of the variables available to us.

Crazy, I thought. *The things we're finding out about on this path to discovery are things we never considered. Things we didn't even know to ask about, but now we're racing headlong down this path, having said yes.* Those things that just showed up during our campaign, most certainly, have changed our course, again and again.

I learned that a vasectomy reversal is a simple outpatient microsurgery procedure performed under local anesthesia, and it requires about a week's recovery time. During the procedure, the surgeon reconnects the vas deferens tubes that carry sperm from the testicle to the semen. There are two methods which can be used to achieve this. In a vasovasostomy, the surgeon sews the ends of each tube back together. There is a more complicated vasoepididymostomy, during which the tubes are attached directly to the epididymis, a small duct at the back of each testicle that holds sperm.

Success rates on reversal and subsequent pregnancy vary by several factors, one of which is the time that has elapsed since the vasectomy. If the procedure was performed less than three years prior, ninety-seven percent of men once again receive sperm in the semen, with a subsequent pregnancy rate of seventy-six percent.[3] From three to eight years, eighty-eight percent sperm and fifty-three percent successful pregnancy. After fifteen years, seventy-one percent sperm and thirty percent pregnancy. Factored into success rates are also the health and age of the father and mother. I was fifty-two at the time, and Nataliya was thirty-eight.

Once the doctor told us about the statistical possibility of getting pregnant, the effects of my age and the number of years since I had the vasectomy hung around my neck like a heavy weight.

And worse, I had been on testosterone therapy for over five years—another deterrent, the consequences of which we were unaware. What we didn't know prior to seeing a urologist is that testosterone therapy stops the pituitary gland from giving the signal to those parts necessary for making natural testosterone, which you must have to make sperm (seed) for the process of getting pregnant. This would be one of the greatest hurdles for us to overcome—to apprehend my seed.

We were making progress in fulfilling the promise, or so we thought. House sold, new school for Tyler, building a new home. And then we visited the urologist.

Before a vasectomy reversal, it is necessary to see if there are any sperm available. In order to check sperm production, the doctor uses a needle inserted into the epididymis to retrieve a sample.

---

[3] https://www.arizona-urology.com/blog/what-is-the-success-rate-for-a-vasectomy-reversal

How can we have a baby who's supposed to come from my seed if there is no seed? Even knowing this, we agreed to move forward in our partnership; we said yes to the promise and started walking down this bumpy road together with thoughts of increasing our progeny. The promise now carried by two. We thought we could manage, but at that time, we did not know that "by my seed" could be more complicated and challenging than we had anticipated. Many other couples find this difficulty waiting for them, too, the further and further they walk down this road, the pathway to discovery.

It was there, at the urologist's office, through multiple meetings over the next four months, that we began to realize the truth of our circumstances. The journey and course on which we were embarking headlong ended at the face of an unclimbable mountain. At first, the guarantee the Frisco doctor provided was awesome: successful reconnection (vasectomy reversal) and assurance that sperm would be flowing...or it's free!

Wow, what a great deal, we thought. Only to discover this didn't apply to me because of the testosterone therapy I was on, which exempted us from any guarantee.

"One's migration into faith's variables," I called it. In other words, faith is the bridge between where I am and the place God is taking me.

One with God and one that holds us captive to outcome, having said yes. And rarely sharing more steps than the one that's before you, trotting with Him. Truly an expedition of faith.

He kept us moving forward one step at a time, and we are thankful for that. But to promise a child will come and not share some of the difficulties that await, and the length of time to get there—yikes!

How to arrive at a place and the peace remains hidden until you fully arrive? God's best waiting on the other side of the hurdle.

We continue to say yes, even when the normal methods no longer work to get us from point A to point B, following Him with each new step, a continued learning process, one keeping us more invested, keeping us moving forward towards the unseen goal He has for us. God gave us grace for the journey. We learned a step-by-step measure of heavenly grace. Grace is not always what people think it is. At times it is the fuel and power to move past the difficulty, down the path to the next step that looks defeating.

We are learning on the fly. The hard facts of our current reality becoming our new reality at the same time, a new kind of normal. In just a few months after having said yes, and only through multiple meetings with many doctors, the hard facts, those bearing down on us, become our new story. Real facts of what difficulty lay before us becoming known.

Dr. J.B.'s instruction to me was this: "You, sir, are going to go off testosterone therapy. To start, you'll begin a twice-a-week regimen of 1 ml shots 5K IU of HCG injection to begin the stimulation, restart your pituitary gland." This was to make natural testosterone instead of the artificial I had been injecting once a week for the last five years. "This should probably do it," he said.

So I asked, "Now why are we doing this?"

"To get sperm flowing again," he said. Then he added, "After one month, we'll check your natural testosterone levels."

Well, I knew they'd be down, way down. I went from a 900 count, down to 215—not a good start. I was tired, edgy, and run-down.

A new normal would now begin to slowly shape our lives. A snail's pace. Like that of a glacier. Moving outward from our center, slowly, cutting through lives, reshaping the old normal into something new over time.

One month later, his office informed me, "You'll need to go one more month on the HCG regimen to bring up those levels." Another month of my being stuck with a needle twice a week.

HCG stands for human chorionic gonadotropin, a hormone produced during pregnancy. Several years ago, people got HCG injections to promote weight loss because it was thought to cause the release of up to 2,500 calories from stored fat.

The process is becoming more intense, and I am getting injections twice a week. A blood sample from me would probably show I was pregnant, because that's the chemical that they look for to tell if a woman is pregnant. And here I am injecting myself weekly with all the stuff—likely to show that I am more pregnant than my wife had I been tested.

After the month had passed, the doctor had me come into his office for a different procedure, one to see if my body was responding to the HCG injections. This procedure was uncomfortable—a needle inserted into the epididymis duct above the testicles, where mature sperm are stored. The stories he shared about other patients' successes gave us hope. Nataliya and I had high expectations for what might be found after the procedure.

The doctor went into the lab to check his findings under a microscope; then he returned to the room where we were and told us, "There were no sperm present."

Seriously? Those words were unbearably difficult to hear.

Expectations dashed against the rocks, gone was the inward hope we had, which was based on the stories he had shared, and we were floundering.

The storms of life now raging against us, finding no shelter, no place to hide.

We were fully exposed to our previous hidden fear. The what-if about the procedure not being successful. Yes, we were heartbroken, to say the least.

Next, the doctor had us come into his office to tell us what our options were, followed by a hint of authority about what to do next.

This was one more step into God's unseen world. We cried inwardly, *This journey, can we do it? Do we have the strength to do it?* It was definitely becoming more difficult the further we went down this path, and yet, we had no inclination that we were just scratching the surface of what complications and frustrations awaited us.

There is something else I want to share with you that threw a wrench into the process for us. My wife received a phone call from her doctor in mid-December, telling her that her lab results from the last Pap smear were irregular—"mild cervical dysplasia," they called it.

We now know there's nothing mild about this news.

Cervical dysplasia describes the abnormal growth of cells on the surface of the cervix. This precancerous condition is caused by the human papillomavirus (HPV), a sexually transmitted infection, or a compromised immune system. An abnormal result such as this is found in one out of ten Pap smears, and the dysplasia often disappears post-pregnancy. It does not mean cancer is present, but does indicate a future possibility.

This kind of news is dislocating to anyone's ear. It certainly can unhinge you from previous hope. So now we must schedule surgery for her to go in and have this taken care of—be given a "clean bill of health," the doctor said, before we could ever become pregnant.

IVF protocol requires that cervical dysplasia be treated before continuing with the procedure. Thankfully, it is dealt with by employing a straightforward laser treatment, which destroys the cells.

Chapter 8

The Goal Still Attainable?

In the beginning of January, we found ourselves back in the urologist's office. "This time the goal is the same goal—to find enough sperm to validate a reversal," the doctor said, followed by, "What we'll do next is continue on the HCG injections for two more months. Then after four months into this, two months longer than expected, and with the shots increased to 1 ml three times a week…that should probably do it."

Two months later, we arrived back at his office with high expectations, having healed from the news we received the last time. And with the aspiration procedure from both sides this time, he said, "We'll definitely find sperm."

Again, after stepping into the other room where the microscope sits waiting, and then coming back into our room, the doctor said, "I can't believe it." After four months in—more time than usual to find what he has in the past, based on his previous findings in others—all he could see under the microscope that day was one lonely sperm.

Needless to say, we were again beside ourselves at these findings. We were left wondering if we could really achieve our goal with the time already spent to find just one. After four months, we were basically at the same place where we started—the big question before us, boldly exclaiming sarcastically, *Where do we go from here? Eight months to find two?*

This would be difficult to hear for almost anyone. We wondered and asked God, *"What have you called us to? Leading us where we find no hope?"*

Allow me to share—if to just reaffirm for myself—this was not just any baby; this was a promised child from God. A promise that I believed to be true when I said yes. A promise God made to my wife. This is what we both believed deep down—we were to have a baby, and it would come from my body, my seed, according to my wife. It is very hard to process thoughts like this, ones with such biblical parallels, especially knowing our Bible speaks of such events.

Abraham, too, was told something similar regarding his seed. Something he almost didn't believe after a time—a similar reaction to the one I was beginning to have.

With all that we were going through during this process, to have the doctor tell us that he's never had a patient who had no sperm, or just one, what were we to think? I'll tell you what we thought. *God can make the impossible possible. A stretch of road we now find ourselves on. Coincidentally, the same road.*

We decided to continue down that same path, the unknown road, believing God. As hard as it was in that moment, we continued to have faith. Confronted with the impossible, and as confused as we were at times, we stayed on the path He had us on, that clandestine course, finding it more and more to be a course of deep privacy as time went on.

Let your eyes look straight ahead; fix your gaze directly before you. (Proverbs 4:25)

God was quietly saying to us, "From now on, this is to stay between you two and no one else." Truly this is what we believed.

Yes, we were tempered to stay quiet and tempted at the same time to share with family and friends—but didn't. It was difficult to remain silent sometimes because of the continuous letdowns. Through the heartache of it all, we continued to feel the best choice was to not risk breaking the hearts of so many others with the constant disappointments. Who could have known that it was going to take years before the promise became a living child?

Who would have stayed the course for 130 weeks of bad news, new challenges, and setbacks? Who would want to listen to that week after week? Even the most supportive people would have become fatigued from holding our hands and helping us carry that load as we walked down that two-and-a-half-year road.

He who has unreliable friends soon comes to ruin, but there is a friend who sticks closer than a brother. (Proverbs 18:24)

I would more than once recall the hymn "What a Friend We Have in Jesus" with comfort and encouragement.

Chapter 9

Believing God in the Midst of Trauma

The promise has been alive in my wife's heart for one year by now. As we're living in our little apartment, our new home is being built with the second bedroom we thought we needed, the second room on the main floor. We are being schooled, both of us having walked with God for some time through a variety of issues in our marriage together.

Believing this promise would prove to be the most difficult thing we ever did—believing God in the midst of trauma. The promise was the primary reason for our move in the first place.

Through and through, we are both praying and trusting Him in this vestige, the residue left on us both from having begun and stayed the course, wearing it like a heavy piece of clothing day in and day out. This step-by-step unfolding fruition hanging off us like an oversized winter coat. Literally wearing the pain, this endeavor, this journey, this however long and bumpy path we must walk down together, alone in our silence. For where else can we go to find the hope we were looking for?

Deep within me, seeds of doubt were produced over time, intermittently creeping into my mind. I could not help myself, thinking, *This guest room awaiting an arrival, this second room on the main floor, desperately needed we thought, would it be a nursery or just an extra room unoccupied most of the time, a promise by God not fulfilled?* How could I think such a thing?

A hard reality to chew on at times. The process of waiting seemingly with no end in sight. As I said, we were being schooled in the multi-divides of God, His unseen world where time is of no consequence. It was quite a ride at times having to battle these thoughts. Feeling naked and exposed, failure parading, to our dismay.

And although it was a thought I wrestled with at times, my wife, too, ended a conversation more than once with, "It will; it will; it will. It must, I declare!"

It became so taxing. Time marching on. An ominous reflection at times for both of us, the mirror on the wall hiding nothing. It occupied my entire soul, and my wife, too, experienced the overload of conscience through trials that just flogged our faith. Looking again in the mirror, seeing myself, and at the same time sensing God's presence so near that if not for Him, I would never have taken another step if He had not given me the strength to do so.

It always came back around in my mind, though—the Holy Spirit reminding me that it will, it will, and it will! The memory of Scripture apprehending my heart, then my hearing, saying to me, "Because God is not a man, that He would lie, or a son of man, that He would change his mind" (Numbers 23:19).

"Yes," I said. "No way will we be defeated!" The Scriptures are true. Affirmed once again, I declared inwardly, *He will do what He has promised…always.* And that's all there is to that.

We must stand on this promise—the promise of God. Only with His help will we be able to handle anything He has spoken—that same power that formed the universe we occupy and live in.

Both of us were exhausted. The arduous times caused tears to fall. We were *choosing to stand with God, His promise, the one He made to both of us after I entered into that promise, having said yes. I must stay strong! Lord, help me!*

Chapter 10

A Change
of Plans

February is upon us, and the plan has changed. Not that the baby won't come from my seed, but it won't be coming through the natural process, through vasectomy reversal. Today, we are introduced to the term "IVF," in vitro fertilization.

A new idea? No, it's been around for decades—but a new path for us, and after many months pursuing the V-reversal. Why? I'm not sure, except to say that God, He knew all of this in advance.

Mid-February and the next step in our adventure takes us to a fertility clinic in Grapevine, Texas, a place recommended by my urologist. Wow, that was a long two-hour meeting, but worth every minute of it. I am reminded in my heart of when the Lord said in Hosea 4:6, "My people perish because of a lack of knowledge." He wasn't mistaken.

We learn that IVF is the process by which the egg and the sperm are fertilized outside of the uterus. Eggs are extracted from the ovaries and fertilized in a laboratory with sperm that has been collected the same day or with sperm that has been collected earlier and frozen until the day they are to be used. The eggs undergo an embryo culture for two to six days and are then transferred to the uterus. More than eight million babies have been born thanks to this and other assisted reproductive technologies (ART)—such as, gamete intrafallopian transfer (GIFT), pronuclear stage tubal transfer (PROST), tubal embryo transfer (TET), and zygote intrafallopian transfer (ZIFT).

In women younger than thirty-five, there is a twenty-one- to thirty-seven-percent chance that the embryo transferred into the uterus this way will result in a viable live birth. That percentage drops, with the age of the mother, to less than one percent in women over forty-four years old. The success rate varies greatly with each study and increases with time as procedures become more refined.

And a whole new direction is before us in the blink of an eye. The bumpy path getting bumpier. *No small thing for any man,* I thought, *this new direction.* One of uncertainty regarding my masculinity, where humility must come forth if another step on the path is to be taken.

So where do we go from here? Many more questions arise because of the new path on which we find ourselves. But not to God—there's no question He's unaware of.

He knew where we would end up from our very beginning. From our first step when we said yes. He knew if we'd choose to keep stepping with Him. He knew all along the ending before the starting point. He remembered my confession—*No small thing...* Now, we'd been delivered to that revelation.

Knowing then the new charge, stretching me as it was, still at times awful thoughts plagued me. I was beginning to get a taste of how it must have been for others who've endured this battle of waiting like Abraham and Sarah in the Bible—another great story of promise and the wait to get there. The promise of a child came to Abraham, seventy-five, and Sarah, sixty-five. They had to wait, and wait, and then wait some more. Abraham was one hundred and Sarah ninety when their promised child, Isaac, was born. Oh, what people take for granted when getting pregnant through the natural course, not all, but most, without much effort.

It would be easy for anyone to give up, especially when they don't have the answers to get them to the next step. Uncertainty causes people's hopes to perish. Feeling defeated, many people give up the plans before them—gone forever because they lacked the knowledge of options that would have helped them. Because of this, I would never fault them for quitting. Pain, anguish, sleep loss, anxiety, and more await most who choose this path to bring a new life into the world.

No, I would never fault any of them for quitting, having gone through it myself. Only the grace of God kept our feet planted on the path all through that arduous process. At times, we fell off the road and into the ditch, battered and bruised, having suffered a true beating.

As Dr. R.C. was going over our case, we learned more than we ever thought we could about how IVF works. We also found out that Nataliya had some fibroids (benign tumors).

"They need to be removed through surgery," her doctor said, if the pregnancy was to have a chance at succeeding.

Just one more thing, I thought, *another surgery.* We were doing again what we were getting used to doing. We were waiting for what's next. Not really knowing what to expect, just as the fibroids had shown up.

Here we are, the end of February. Nataliya has gone in for blood work again for the appointment she'll have next week.

• • •

It is now the first week of March. This appointment is to verify the condition of Nataliya's uterus for carrying our child. For me, it looks like I will undergo one more month of HCG treatment before my surgery for sperm extraction—hoping we are successful.

Her appointment went well this time. It's a first for me, looking at the inside of a uterus through ultrasound—and although two fibroids were present and one polyp—hmm, looks like more stuff to deal with and, of course, more waiting. Hence, not really knowing what's next, but just showing up.

• • •

I've since made my appointment for April 8, 2015—one year, four months from the genesis, when the promise was placed in my wife's heart. The appointment for the biopsy of my right testicle. They'll be taking a few pieces out, about "one-tenth the size of a small fingertip," he said.

• • •

Wow, how time flies; today's the 8th, and there's a multitude of voices going through my head. Some doubting. Others speaking. Those flybys making suggestions about the what-ifs. To defuse that noise—please, anything to take my mind off of it—I took the dog to the dog run at our apartment before we left for the hospital. It was five o'clock in the morning. There, I found myself quieted, beginning to praise God for the adventure of the day.

Anxious, though, not knowing what will happen. Just one quiet moment was all I needed in order to take the next step.

But more serious now, interrupting me, it seemed to be the wave of words once again on the walk back to the apartment. The what-ifs, they just kept coming into my mind—a flood of deep water, and I was just trying to stay afloat on dry land. It was difficult walking back to the apartment.

Then in a moment, that unruly thought, the attack the enemy had become so good at planting—doubt—it was seized and taken captive by a more powerful thought. Ironically, one that *gently* came in, in the midst of this storm I was drowning in. Instead of "what if," it became "what's next," as this question seemed to have dominated our thoughts during our peregrination through the door of one doctor's office after the next. This confused us somewhat in the moment, as if "what's next" was better somehow in this continuance,, this step-by-step, frustrating expedition we had been on since we said yes.

What will we do next? I mean, after today, I thought—meaning, if things didn't work out for us. *What's next after all that we've gone through to get to this place?*

These were the kind of thoughts I was having. Before we left for the surgery center that morning, my wife reaffirmed me. She anointed my head with oil, calling out in me the truth of what God says about me in His word. She reminded me that I am a child of God, and His plan for me is to not harm me but to give me hope and a future. That declaration alone is what made it better; it calmed the storm within.

Chapter 11

Ready

We're ready to go see my doctor, walking through one more door of uncertainty.

We had no idea what was going to be found that day with the biopsy, especially after what happened before. The hope was for more than one sperm. The thought going through both of our minds was, *Please be more this time.*

We were overjoyed when our doctor came into the room and told us that he not only found good sperm, but that he found many! We couldn't have been more relieved with the news.

The sperm were frozen for the future. We were finally there, reassured, a new place on the path. Rescue had found us! It was a very sobering day for both of us.

•••

Almost seven months have gone by, and God's promise is still persuading both of us to stay the course, keeping us safe in the plan He has for us.

We couldn't have been more thankful in that moment. We could breathe and had a newfound hope. We rested in that moment, gaining strength for whatever would be next on our path.

The biopsy plug harvested that day was taken to the lab. It is there that they retrieved the sperm we needed, processing them for freezing, and for what we thought we'd do later.

Chapter 12

Launch

The countdown is on. It is the now the 16th of May. Nataliya goes in on the 21st to have the fibroids removed. My participation in this journey began back in July of 2014, and she has carried this promise around since the beginning of 2014. At times it seems as though we are witnessing a countdown to…what? The unknown. Something that's out there, somewhere, maybe to arrive one day.

There is hope within us that differs from other couples who just become pregnant, those who simply find out that they are and nine months later deliver in the usual way. But for our journey, God straightens the path before us. He nourishes our hope day in and day out, giving us strength. He levels mountains and fills valleys, making a level plane where I can see clearly again.

I say again to myself, I can, and it will*! Followed by,* Blessed be my Lord for the view He's given me. It is only with His help that I am able to see beyond the current struggle. *We both glance forward unto the promised child. We inwardly parade the grace that has been given to us.*

In our hearts, strangely, it felt as if we were already pregnant. For they were the tangible words we both needed and found—"I can" and "it will"! Only God, could have made available the strength we needed that day to keep stepping forward on the path He had chosen for us. So again we wait, but not in vain—standing on hope—that was the grace given to us that day.

Proven

God has proven to us that, deep inside both of us, He's very present in these moments of waiting. These times when our character is being tried, yet built at the same time into that which He desires. Waiting for the 21st with hope. It's a hope in knowing that in approximately three months, we could be pregnant. And have the fullness of His desired intent growing inside her womb. We continue to wait for the promise that was given to us.

The 21st of May is here. The procedure went well. Our doctor said, "The baby's home"—meaning, in the womb—"and ready to go."

So we wait again, waiting as we've gotten used to—holding out a hope that we're now used to as well. One thing's for sure—waiting on God's promise is far different than waiting for tomorrow's daylight or anything else we expect to come.

Tomorrow has arrived so many times before just as we were convinced it would, without much thought. The sun continues to rise, and we expect tomorrow's daylight, just like we expect our next breath as a God-given freedom. Waiting on God's promise consumes our most personal space, inner workings, and with the prompting of hope as fuel, it incites an intense longing. God has indeed placed within us, not just the promise, but this longing to wait on Him, waiting with faith that His promise will arrive one day. Yes, far different than believing tomorrow's daylight will come.

Yes. I must enthusiastically say yes because of where we've already walked with Him, for He is our God. He is our grace. He is our cover! One must stay inclined to this outcome, or nothing more could have fit into our lives, our current moments, without some kind of permanent mental damage to us.

Chapter 14

On the Road Again

It's time for the next step through another door. On June 19th, Nataliya goes in to have her blood drawn again. If the numbers that we're looking for, hormonewise, are good, they will tell us if eggs are present in her ovaries.

Our doctor likes what she sees—thank goodness—and she tells us that the numbers are good for the production of eggs!

The next step is to start drug-stimulation therapy—the remedial therapeutics that go hand in hand with IVF, quickly arousing the ovaries to produce.

The most wonderful part—we've been given a tentative date for egg retrieval—July 28th. This date is one year from the time Nataliya brought me the revelation she received. She spoke it out to me, and now, one and half years after her vision—the Lord's promise of a child—we are now really on our way.

We continue to pray for healthy eggs. But prior to the egg retrieval, we'll have to go and see Nataliya's doctor one more time to be sure her fibroids are all gone.

I'm very aware, through the whole process of IVF, that many of the things that we pray for, many of the hopes my wife and I have, are the kinds of things that most people would never pray about during the natural process of getting pregnant. They are the kinds of things that many people take for granted.

Truly, this has been an amazing adventure, though. It has been taxing beyond what many people could comprehend. The difficulties are something that cannot be understood by anyone who hasn't gone through IVF. Most people will never know the great struggle of going down this path.

Chapter 15

One More Door

On the last visit to Nataliya's doctor, we again received some news that we were hoping to be different. Sadly, we were told another fibroid is pressed into the uterine cavity. The future embryo's home is possibly compromised, which would most certainly complicate a pregnancy. Inwardly, gut-wrenchingly, objectionably, I protest.

Regardless, Nataliya will have to go through fibroid surgery once again. Another grievous setback.

We are waiting again with hopes of an egg retrieval in late August. We are beginning to see a pattern emerge. We will not allow the enemy—defeat—to void God's promise. We will not succumb to the defeat of such continuous trials, which would stop many in their tracks. We continue to brace ourselves for what's next on this path to the unknown.

I've learned that time can sometimes be your comforter. Having a future date to focus on, a possible date for what you've been waiting for…hoping for…brings a new confidence and an increased desire at times.

We hope while holding the hand of faith. Our faith is strengthened during the wait. We continue to walk towards a hope that is real. A hope that's becoming manifest. However, with this date given to us, you know what that means—the possibility of becoming pregnant by the first week of September. We both say yes to that!

•••

The fibroid-removal procedure went very well. The doctor was able to get the whole fibroid out this time. Last time, she was only able to remove part of a fibroid. As thorough as my wife's doctor is, I'm sure she'll be looking inside the cavity again just to be sure. We continue to pray for a clean sweep next time. To hope for no more return trips to the surgery room.

The date is now July 20th, one year from the time Nataliya returned from MPC the second time—six months after the genesis of God's promise and the new path He brought her to. His vision given to her—the promise of having a child with me. How life altering it's been.

It's hard to believe what we've gone through so far. Three surgeries for Nataliya, two aspirations for me, and one biopsy-plug retrieval from my right testicle.

And now, I have just found out that there is another surgery I will need in order to retrieve fresh specimens. The frozen sperm is only used as a backup if none can be found on the day of fertilization. Prompting my next statement, "You mean I have to go through this biopsy again, #*%&@!?"

I put that aside. I think we are really getting close now, and we're both very excited. We remember that God's ways are not our ways, nor is His timing the same as ours. This is a hard lesson we are learning, one that God is growing us through together. Not that we haven't walked with God through other difficulties, but we are being reminded, and reminded again, that His ways are far different than ours. That's the hard lesson that can only be taught through time, the very thing we have fought through to get to where we are.

•••

Here we are in late August. Nataliya has been scheduled to begin Luteal Lupron, one of the drug options prescribed to women as part of the IVF protocol. Normally, the ovaries release one egg per cycle. The goal of retrieval is to secure 10–18 eggs to optimize the chances of success. Drugs increase egg production, therefore IVF success rates.

But we are confronted with another problem. The doctor tells us that Nataliya now has a cyst on her ovary, which must subside prior to starting the Lupron, which is scheduled to begin within the next ten days. Otherwise, those stimulation meds will contribute to the growth of the cyst.

So we pray, just like we've been praying, many times during the day—every day. We just keep on stepping as He continues to lead us.

Chapter 16

Praying

*Okay, both kinds of news. We're unsure what to do next. This has been a
long journey for us and can be for many other couples on this path, where
there is constantly a turn to the right, another to the left, one more to the
right. Through this, we have learned more about trusting Him and about
His skills that guide us, navigate for us, and direct us. Constantly, over and
under, through and around. We know…we have faith…that we'll be okay,
whichever way the path turns.*

This type of schooling alters one's life more and more, and
trust must be found to continue.

• • •

*The next turn, the next news, is that Nataliya's cyst has subsided. Praise!
Now it is manageable for the stimulation meds.*

*In the same phone call…turn again. Her estrogen levels are too high to
move forward with the stimulation.*

The emotional roller coaster we were on was hard to put into words, except one—"exhausting"! The type of exhaustion known only to those on the confusing path of IVF.

If it isn't one thing, it's certainly been another (crying), or something other than another, and another, seemingly a never-ending story for us. Our prayer has been and continues to be that mature, healthy eggs are found, and only God knows that timing.

We are told that we'll have to wait again. What's next? The same story continues. So now we wait until her cycle next month. Afterwards, if all looks good, then stimulation meds will begin. We wait, and we wait.

Chapter 17

Praying More!

How much prayer is enough? If prayer is a conversation with God, but no answers are found yet, and longing continues for the promised outcome, then one should continue the conversation as if one is learning to walk on a new road. Likely a road never walked down before. God holding one's hands, never letting go through the ups and downs, unders and overs, arounds and abouts, as we give thanks and do it all over again.

Nataliya will begin her new cycle on October 13th. And yes, still in the year 2015. We are now told by our doctor that, if we move forward aggressively with the stimulation meds, then we'll be retrieving eggs by the 26th of October, barring any more complications.

This completely takes us by surprise since the process feels as if it had been taking forever. Finally, our doctor is setting us up to harvest eggs about five weeks after Nataliya's cycle begins.

This date, however, is the day we are scheduled to move from the apartment to our new house. The home with the second room on the main floor, and we're not even pregnant yet. The moving company tells us that they are unable to change the date for our move.

Again, conflict. Luckily, our doctor can provide birth control pills, which would draw things out a bit until after the move, kind of like placing the eggs in a holding pattern.

It seems counterproductive to use birth control pills as part of a protocol to get pregnant, doesn't it? We thought so, too, until it was explained to us. Turns out, it is a very common practice. To be more accurate, I will quote a blog I came across.

> *First, in a normal menstrual cycle multiple follicles (which contain the eggs) begin to grow, but then one follicle becomes dominant and grows faster than the rest, and the remaining follicles stop progressing. In an IVF cycle, though, we want as many follicles as possible to grow. By taking birth control pills before starting the ovarian stimulation medications, the follicles are more likely to grow at a similar rate. This leads to a greater number of follicles being mature at the same time, and therefore increases the number of eggs that are retrieved. Using birth control pills also allows the fertility clinic to effectively schedule retrievals.[4]*

Our new date for egg retrieval and fertilization is now set for November 17th.

We wait on the promise set in the timing of God's providence. There is no safer place as He is teaching us more about who He is in our lives.

•••

November 17th comes with another setback, another cyst on Nataliya's right ovary.

---

[4] https://www.inviafertility.com/blog/use-of-birth-control-pills-in-ivf-process

However, the doctor tells us that we're still going to try to use the eggs we currently have, but not harvested yet—crazy. Tricking and manipulating my wife's body—it is astonishing that they can do such things. She will have to go into outpatient surgery once again and have the cyst drained. Followed by birth control pills again to suppress.

How many surgeries now? I've lost count. We suspect egg retrieval will be sometime around the end of November—maybe. One more time around the mountain, it seems.

And that word again—"exhausting." A heavy word. A weight found hidden for most in the world of IVF debacles. A word buried in life's most difficult times, and a word that doesn't let go until you're through the trauma, exhumed, and on to something else. Restored to the path again for what's next. The up and down, around and over we are delivered to once again.

A storm that's all too real. Not to harm, but a storm that's to clear the way before us as we're being led through it.

•••

It's now December 2nd. We have once again been given some sad news. Another cyst problem. One biting us in the #@&*, and we're dealing with it. #$%$*!

We are now having to wait for an entire cycle again, another trip around the mountain, when maybe, just maybe, we'll be able to start stimulation sometime around December 25th.

Emotionally, a biting wait. A debilitating "weight." An unfamiliar weariness weighing on both our shoulders now. Not just a winter coat, but a wet winter coat. A brutality that seemingly won't let up. We are tired of getting bad news, but He has shown us it is never more than we can handle. We find a strength living within that is not of ourselves.

A quote I read somewhere about IVF is very fitting to our situation.

> *What most people don't, and will likely never, fully under-stand, not unless they go through IVF. It is the amazing, stressful, chaotic, painful, surprising, depressing, confusing, inspirational journey that women (and men) undergoing IVF treatments embark on...and I have only scratched the surface on the scope of emotion.*

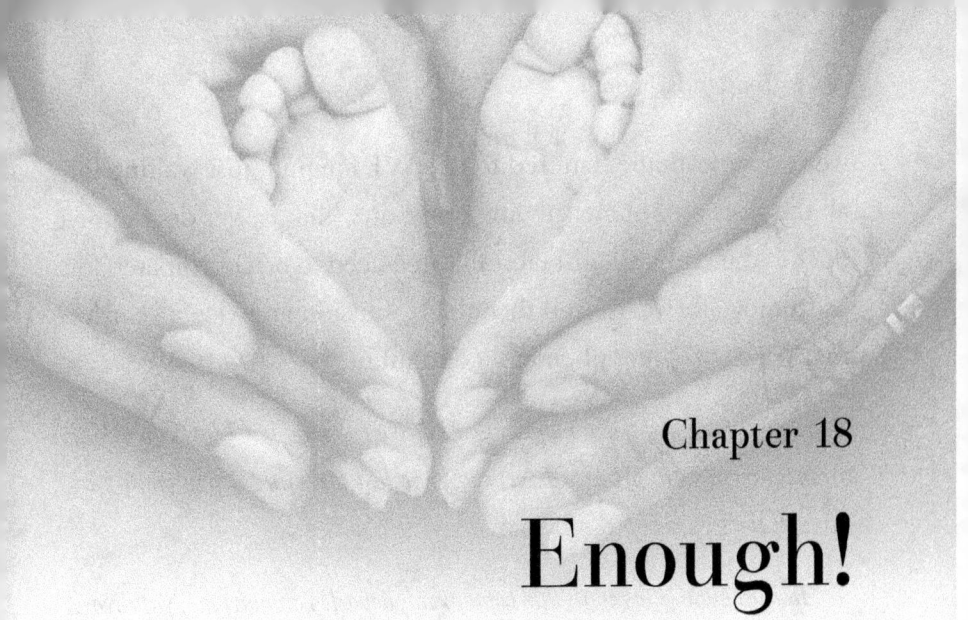

Chapter 18

Enough!

All right already! Yes, it's now December 29th. One and a half weeks ago, Nataliya had another sonogram, which was good, no cyst—but wait, wait for it...........................we now have a supposed polyp problem again.

Really?! I could just scream. But I don't, because that is what maturity has brought me—silent acceptance. Begrudging, but silent. So we schedule another minor surgery for her in a few days.

•••

Well, it turned out to be nothing; still, it meant another trip to the OR. And time ambles on, continuing to flee.

And the cost to many who go through this IVF theorem existence—money, patience, time—are all diagnostics of an IVF life. You will test positive to all three and be forced to live life as you wait, delivered to the abyss, left to watch from the background.

Time's grip, an ephemeral catch to those found in IVF's paradigm. Many can only watch as it's slipping away. Therefore, we're symptomatic, fettered to this IVF enigma, just waiting for all the stars and planets to line up again—that is, her doctor, my doctor, the embryologist lab. All three need to be coordinated for us to move forward. And the lab? It shuts down twice a year for maintenance—an ephemeral continuum.

I know there are a few more things I'd like to share, but I just can't think of them right now because I seem to have lost my mind a few steps back through the trauma of it all.

To help both of us with this timing/lab debacle conundrum, Nataliya is on birth control for another 20 days, attempting to salvage these eggs again. Praying some more, we wait. Waiting becomes a life-form of its own. One in our home, one at work, everywhere we are, and it lives. Sometimes feeding it. Other times, feeding it too much as time's march advances.

•••

Twenty days have now passed by. We spent yesterday morning at her doctor's office in Grapevine. Having gone through the twentieth or so transvaginal sonogram, waiting the last seven months because of a cyst (twice), a polyp (once, and possibly twice as the second surgery was necessary), a fibroid (twice), a blood clot, another cyst, the lab shutting down, or something else, estrogen levels not cooperating.

•••

We are moving forward with stimulation, starting today, January 15ᵗʰ, 2016. And yes, right at two years from Nataliya's first conception when the Lord spoke to her heart saying, "Who made the choice when you said you were done having children? Was that Me—God—or you who made that choice without Me?"

Our egg retrieval is set for January 27th. Hallelujah! Again, grateful for this step-by-step walk of faith, and no other way could we have arrived without the Lord's constant intervention pushing us forward.

Without His help, I would have given up long ago. If all this were known up-front, most people would probably choose not to walk down this road, knowing all the heartache and all that goes along with it. Would not say yes to something so out of their control. IVF is a solitary journey of the heart for many, where time is not their comforter, but their contender.

Chapter 19

'A More Real Time'

Today marks five days into the stimulation. We have a doctor's appointment for another sonogram. Getting a sonogram is kind of like going on a blind date. You can wish and guess all you want, but you really have no idea what is going to happen until you get there. An arrangement in our lives, lately set by others. Leaving us with a fully nourished anxiety. Until then, both of us feel like we're standing on the edge of a chasm with no bottom, leaning over the edge, to see what cannot be seen.

What might we see today? A question we have anxiously asked many times, and are always surprised by the answer. What will it be today? A cyst, a fibroid, a polyp? Maybe a blood clot. Maybe none of the above, but something new?

At first, it looked like there were more cysts, but to our surprise, the doctor said, "What you are seeing on the screen, those are all follicles, and likely with eggs, getting bigger, growing Exactly what we want to see."

We were inflated with joy to hear such a report! We could breathe again. A sigh of relief poured from us. Tomorrow was now today, and the news was good this time.

Chapter 20

One Week Later

We left the house at 5:30 a.m., before the sun was up, to make our 6:00 a.m. appointment. The doctor has dictated my wardrobe for the day: tight shorts and a tight T-shirt with a top pocket. I dressed on the assumption he meant for me to wear a bit more than that, so added a pair of jeans and an oxford-cloth shirt on top.

We dropped Nataliya at the hospital. You would think I could be with her as they prep her for the egg-retrieval procedure. But no, that would have been way too simple.

Instead, I excitedly tell Nataliya goodbye—this could be the day!—get back in the car, park at the building across the street, and head inside for my second testicular biopsy. This procedure can be used in a number of situations: to detect the nature of a lump in the testicles, to detect a cause of infertility, and in my case, to extract fresh sperm for the embryologist to use in the procedure that will take place just moments from now.

There are a variety of ways to perform this procedure. A percutaneous biopsy uses a needle for extraction. Some doctors perform an open biopsy, which means a tiny cut with a stitch or two to close the incision. For mine, an incision was made. A spring-loaded device was inserted, snapped shut very quickly to capture the plug containing the sperm, and then removed. Thank goodness, it all happens pretty fast.

The doctor had instructed me to wear tight shorts so that I could pack them with ice to prevent swelling. And the tight shirt? That is so I can place the biopsy plastic vial, which measures about two inches long and three-eighths of an inch across, in my pocket, keeping it close to my chest and warm while I make the trip back across the street.

So I jog to my car, one hand holding my Tommy Johns packed with ice, the other hand holding the vial securely in my pocket. I hop into the car, put it in gear, negotiate four lanes of traffic, and search for a parking space to make it back to Nataliya.

Now, you don't just hand off the specimen tube to someone who goes in the back room and pours it into a petri dish. No, that specimen is given to an embryologist; then it is washed and placed into a solution that emulates the fluid found in the fallopian tubes.

While I was getting my biopsy, Nataliya was prepped and wheeled into a room like an OR to undergo retrieval of the mature eggs. A needle is inserted through the side of the vaginal wall, into the ovary, and then into the follicles within that have eggs waiting to be extracted; each follicle bears one egg. Only after extraction, and through the use of a microscope, can the embryologist know whether they've actually retrieved the egg from inside the follicle. Our hope is that at least eight follicles have eggs in them.

•••

Finally, this is really happening. Nataliya is being wheeled back to the room where I am anxiously waiting. Her doctor enters the room and tells us, "Out of the eight follicles she had, they were able to retrieve six good eggs."

Wow! With that said, the embryologist told us exactly what we were hoping to hear next—they are mature eggs.

Is this is really happening? The fertilization of eggs? We're here! We're finally here! That thought wins the day.

The sperm is injected into the egg. Keep in mind what a miracle this is. An egg so small that you can only see it with a microscope, and a needle no bigger than a fine human hair, and they're being used to inject one sperm into one egg to be fertilized. Amazing! Then the watch-and-wait begins.

The Next Day...

Nataliya and I are sitting in the kitchen. The phone rests on the table between us; we have the embryologist on speaker. She is going to review the fertilization report with us.

Each day, the embryologist watches the cells multiply in the fertilized eggs. If they are healthy embryos, they'll just keep multiplying—32, 64, 128—further multiplying. The nurse also calls to check on how Nataliya is feeling, review the medications she will begin, and schedule a tentative time for embryo transfer.

It's good news! She tells us that they were able to fertilize five of the six eggs, but that only three mature specimens are going to be suitable for the transfer that will happen in three days.

Transfer Day...

Another early morning at the hospital. The embryologist enters the office with one four-by-six picture of three embryos, and we get to choose which two fertilized eggs to transfer into the uterus. Although there is not a great deal of difference in their appearance—other than some are round, while others are oblong—the clinic will not choose for you; the choice is yours so that you can't blame them for failure.

We could have elected to transfer all three, but no, one will stay behind. By day six, hopefully, the one left behind will be doing well enough to be frozen for another time if these two are not successful. We're left to wonder what we may decide to do with it in the future. A frozen embryo will last indefinitely.

A younger person would probably choose to transfer only one fertilized egg because of the likelihood that they would both split, resulting in four children. Older parents frequently decide to transfer two, increasing the chance of a successful pregnancy. If you were using the donor eggs of a younger woman, you would probably only choose to transfer one.

As soon as we choose the two embryos, Nataliya is ready to go through the procedure to have them transferred to her uterus. She is given Valium to relax the uterus, and the whole procedure takes about ten minutes.

An interesting sidenote: the embryos are drawn up into a small tube with a bulb resting in the hand of the doctor, who squeezes it when he sees a location in the uterus that looks right. All of this is being watched on a sonogram screen. What is interesting is that once the bulb is squeezed, forcing the embryos out, there is a little flash of light at the end of the tube that cannot be explained. Afterwards, each embryo searches for the place it will begin its journey. When withdrawn, the device is handed back to the embryologist, who verifies there is nothing left in the tube.

After a little rest, we go home and wait. Nataliya will take it easy the rest of the day while the embryos nestle into the uterus wall.

Now we have a real chance. In a deeper sense, our new growth recognition, this tour de force driving us, a defined perception: A particularly adroit maneuver or technique in handling a difficult situation. One we've continued to find ourselves in, and most certainly found more than not. Learning to do through such extremes, and far more, we wait, trusting God for what's next. For He has been our strength through it all!

Oh yes, you shaped me first inside, then out; you formed me in my mother's womb. (Psalms 139:13)

Chapter 21

Onward

We must wait nine days from the date of transfer to take a blood test to find out if we're pregnant. We pray and wait. With the waiting comes anxiety and excitement.

On day five, we receive a call telling us that the embryo left in the lab has stopped growing the way he or she should in order to be frozen.

This was a sad day for both of us. Losing that embryo means our chances have been decreased. The heartache is revisiting us, teaming with a rent now left on our souls. Tears must fall and did. Who'd of ever thought that one would grieve so much over one so small, one that's hidden out of sight in the quantum dwelling place.

Right now, we're reeling, sojourning in the place of woe, waiting to find out if we're pregnant. It's been a difficult wait after nineteen months—and over two years for Nataliya—not only demanding, but the problematic travail that has continued to plague us physically through and through. The sleepless battering one endures walking down this path. More so, those great difficulties upon one's soul, the abrasions cast unforgivingly through the trauma, through the wait and loss of it all.

It is a very difficult emotion for many people who dare to walk this path to put into words, I suspect. Navigating such deep waters at times and failing again. How does one keep going?

• • •

Today's the day. It is 7:20 Tuesday morning, February 9, 2016. Over two years from the genesis, the life that was spoken into my wife's heart. We find ourselves at the accumulative crossroads this day. Nataliya goes in for her blood test at 9:00 a.m. to see if she's pregnant. From there, we wait for the phone call.

• • •

We just received the call at 3:15 this afternoon. All I can say at this time is that I can't talk right now. My stomach is in knots, too painful to breathe. Our worst fear came true; tears must fall once again. The heartache, just unbearable.

Tears fell for both of us that day as we propped each other up, balancing the failure we were enduring. The days that followed washed our pain and grief away, but not so quickly. More like, smeared it around as we remembered being told, "You're not pregnant."

It was raw and painful for us—as it is for the many who endure this discovery on their IVF journey—a great sadness befell us that day.

Chapter 22

To Move
One Forward

It's been one week since we got the news, and tears are still falling without warning, regardless of who's present. To help us process the loss, we went to the store and picked out three balloons. One that read, "It's a Boy"; another, "It's a Girl"; and still another, "It's a Boy or a Girl," for the embryo that didn't live past day five.

We took the balloons into our backyard that evening, prayed over them as we let them go, and knew one day that we'd see all three of them in heaven. It was a moment of therapy for us. We never wanted anyone else to endure this sadness, but knew nonetheless that it would find others on their journeys of IVF failure. I know better now the risk on the path, one we were called to walk. Experiencing loss as we never had before, we wept together that evening.

Chapter 23

On the Path Again

It would seem our focus again is on what's next. In a few weeks, we'll endure another consultation with Nataliya's doctor, R.C., to see in which direction we'll be stepping. No, we haven't given up; we're just stepping out of the numbness. In one way, it's like learning to walk all over again. Trusting that God is showing Himself to us in our plight. Even in this, His plan for us, it is still to fulfill the promise He made to my wife, then to me as I stood with her upon my yes.

For where else could we go, having come so far? We know He is faithful, regardless of what we see before us. This is what He is teaching us. He schools us further into a lifetime of trusting Him, through this moment in time, walking on a path that few are given the privilege to navigate. The promised calling for one to go forth, following that call, being consumed just walking with Him. The sharp edges, we now see we are being polished in every way, it seems. Experiencing 2 Corinthians 4:8–9, "we are afflicted in every way, but not crushed; perplexed, but not driven to despair; persecuted, but not forsaken; struck down, but not destroyed." And through all this, the promise is still alive within us. Not knowing what lies ahead, yet trusting God in ways we never could before, because of the path we just walked down together.

•••

The other day, we had our consultation with the doctor, and we had many questions we wanted to get sorted out. We've been processing what our other options might be. It was suggested, with the hint of being advised, that "if you can afford to do IVF one more time, maybe you should consider donor eggs."

For us, since Nataliya's promise was not confined to her eggs, this option was certainly one that we were considering. Do we go through one more cycle of IVF? Or double the cost to use donor eggs? Wow. Then, do we use my sperm with those eggs, or do we use donor sperm? So many options we didn't even consider before, not knowing. Feeling overwhelmed again.

Her eggs and my seed—that's what we wanted most. It is difficult to choose and be certain of that choice—a new hardship to maneuver through. But God, showing us our hidden desire, He most certainly moved us. Directing our feet onto the path of His desire, which, by the way, was our desire, one He placed in both of us.

So many questions to digest. Assuredly not wanting to experience that pain all over again, ever. But knowing the reality now, good and well, exactly what could happen if we choose that direction one more time.

We were finding ourselves on that path again. And of what could be our despair? Only He knew.

So to the path again. The choice we wanted was made. It was really a choice that just came about like a natural order. Choosing things we want—or, better said, things we believed God wanted for us—His plan unfolding. The choice we made was the same as we did in the beginning. We chose Nataliya's eggs and my seed.

• • •

Now finding ourselves five weeks after the loss and our balloon ceremony, believe it or not, here we are again stimulating with the transfer to occur within two weeks, and with our own eggs and sperm—amazing!

What's next, Lord? An obvious question we ask ourselves. Will it turn out the same? Treading in deep water, we wait as before. Waiting with a very real concern on our minds, our hearts having endured the worst. But we moved off that line of thinking, pursuing instead what God had started in us afresh. Praying all the way. Only God knows. He is the only one who knows our future. So the time invested in Him through this process, waiting one more time in hope—a needed necessity to ground us in our pursuit.

• • •

We are now nine days into the stimulation, this Sunday, March 20th. It looks like we'll be doing the retrieval Wednesday, the 23rd. With great hope, we'll be transferring two healthy, three- to five-day-old embryos either on the 26th or 28th. What an exhausting spoken thing, but a completely worthwhile journey. We have learned so much.

We have grown in ways we never could have, had we not said yes to God and pursued the course on which He placed us. A path we probably would never have chosen if we'd really known the emotional, physical, and most certainly monetary cost. Yet

God knew all of this before we said yes to any of it. He provided what was needed to get us there, and through it. He knew it all.

• • •

Today is Wednesday the 23rd, and we're at the hospital for the retrieval. We were told that there may only be four eggs today, based on the follicles they saw. As my wife was rolled back into the room, I pondered, What possibility might befall us today?

Her doctor came in a few minutes afterwards, giving us the news. "We have six eggs!"

Such great news to hear. What we're hoping for now is for all six to be healthy enough for fertilization, to make it to day five. Sojourning in hope until tomorrow. What the chances were for these little ones we did not know.

Chapter 24

A Very Special Easter Egg

It's been four days since the retrieval, and it is Easter week. This day is significant because of the vision that my wife had two years and three months ago, attending the MPC conference in Wheaten, where she received the revelation of "a beautiful, multicolored Easter egg" with a baby inside.

Little Treasures

We have now four healthy embryos, we are told! All four doing fine on day three. We are so happy! As we've learned from our previous walk, a lot can happen in one day with these little ones, those that live in the secret place, the quantum dwelling place.

•••

Waiting for day five to get here, we're a bit nervous. We may decide to transfer now, or freeze them all and transfer later. And the rub, not knowing if they'll even make it that long, based on what happened last time. The what-ifs that didn't even have time to set in before we got the news.

•••

So wonderful! We're not used to getting good news on this journey of ours. Always something defeating us, it seems. This long, hard process of IVF, a treacherous road at times. On day five, not only were we able to transfer two healthy embryos, but on day six, we were able to freeze the other two for future use if not successful this time! Dumbfounded at the reversal, at having a real chance, better than previously.

•••

Waiting for those nine days to pass to find out if we're pregnant. We wait.

Earlier today, I was getting ready to write about our experience thus far, but changed my mind. If I had written, it would have been about how discouraged we have been over the last three days of taking pregnancy tests. Tests that were negative. Even this morning on day eight, after the transfer, we're still showing negative. Our hearts are leading us astray based on past failures. Our souls tender, bruised, we wait..

•••

I'm glad I didn't write until now. Because Nataliya took another pregnancy test around 10:00 a.m. Three tests that were all positive! Very surreal. Weeping. Tears of joy fall this time.

Teetering away from sorrow that day, we laughed.

The next day, we went for the blood test to confirm our findings. Yes! We are indeed pregnant!

Surprisingly, what we didn't expect to hear is that, in the IVF world, we are further along than we thought. We are four weeks pregnant already.

Over the next three or four weeks, we were expecting to hear a heartbeat—so exciting, new life teeming.

The longing of our hearts fulfilled. Our past traumas dissipate. We call her by her name—Abigail.

Chapter 25

Five Months Along

At around five months pregnant, Nataliya woke me up one morning, telling me, "I think I'm having labor pains, and I need to go to the emergency room."

In a normal pregnancy, the umbilical cord "is attached to the fetus at the belly button and consists of two arteries and a vein surrounded by protective tissue. It embeds itself into the center of the placenta, which is in turn latched on to the interior of the mother's uterus."[5]

With a velamentous cord insertion (VCI), "the umbilical blood vessels insert into the amniotic sac instead of the placenta."[6]

---

[5] https://www.verywellfamily.com/velamentous-cord-2371665

[6] https://www.verywellfamily.com/velamentous-cord-2371665

One of the complications of velamentous cord insertion is the possibility of going into labor early. Having this condition through pregnancy does set one on edge. A rare and dangerous condition occurring in less than half a percent of all pregnancies, it can result in fetal and maternal blood loss at delivery.

With medication, the doctors at the hospital were able to stop the labor, and Nataliya was able to come home the next day. We thought that getting pregnant would end those disappointments anchored to all the yesterdays, the traumas that we'd endured. But then we had something new to worry about—trying to *stay* pregnant.

It felt like an open wound that wouldn't heal, knowing that, for the next four months, much could go wrong because of the velamentous cord insertion. Nataliya's doctor informed us that, in some cases, a cesarean-section delivery is necessary as early as at thirty-five weeks of gestation, in cases when the blood vessels are found near the cervix. A C-section avoids going through the labor process, which might end up with a stillbirth because of a rupture and the rapid loss of blood. Yes, we had a whole new set of worries consuming us.

There was still a small chance that we could have a vaginal birth, with the baby descending naturally, with the hope of the cord moving to the side a little.

Chapter 26

I Asked Them to Pray

I remember it as if it were yesterday—standing in the birthing room when Nataliya's doctor announced that she was running across town and would be back in thirty minutes.

A nurse made Nataliya more comfortable by placing a two-foot-wide inflated ball between Nataliya's legs, saying that it might help the baby descend farther, making labor easier. I walked out of the room to get something to drink, and a few minutes later when I returned, I instantly noticed a large puddle of blood on the floor under the bed. I looked up at Nataliya in horror as I saw that the bed was soaked with blood too. I yelled for the nurse. The doctor was still not back as they rushed Nataliya out of the room and into the OR.

Left alone and frightened in the room, just staring at the large pool of blood, I began calling our family and friends, crying as I asked them to pray for the lives of Nataliya and our unborn child. I was scared, not knowing if my wife and baby would make it.

After what seemed like forever, a nurse came in and handed me a set of scrubs, saying, "Hurry, put these on." The staff had been busy moving another woman out of the OR to allow Nataliya to be rolled in for this emergency. The nurse ushered me into the OR, which was thankfully located right next door.

As I pushed through the door, I had no idea what to expect, the staff telling me nothing. To my surprise, a nurse placed our baby girl into my arms. I held her gently to my chest and looked over at the exhausted Nataliya. Even having lost two liters of blood, she was doing remarkably well, and even looked up at me and smiled while the nurses tended to her.

The next day, we were back in our room at the hospital and awestruck, as new parents usually are. As I sat in a chair, Nataliya and the baby sleeping, I collected my thoughts. *What an incredible journey this has been.* Very few things, if any, along the way went as planned, but here we were, on the other side of the hurdle God set for us, God's best found that day, safe from all that plagued us. His promise perfect in every way. Thank you, Lord, for being the promise keeper we discovered You to be. Our lives forever changed simply by saying yes.

Chapter 27

A Quiverful–Two Years Later

The joy and heartache of possibility. The what-ifs finally stifled. We had two frozen embryos left from our second IVF round. The thought of another child lingered somewhere within us—a thought that began to thaw, seemingly becoming a possibility in our minds as time passed.

We needed to be good stewards with what we had in our possession in this life—the two frozen embryos that were left from our second IVF round with Abigail. *What should we do with them?*

Remembering the vision I had before Abigail was even conceived—walking down the hallway, holding the hands of two small children—both of our hearts were moved again with the desire to increase our family. Our daughter was two years old now; would we attempt to step again onto the path that brought so much trauma before?

Questions bombarding us: Were we willing to relive all that we had endured before? Were we willing to go through that again, considering everything we had learned in the process? Did we want to get this engine started again?

Do I/we have the stamina for this? Do we want to endure the what-ifs one more time? I think so.

Now, it would seem, Nataliya was in the position of believing, not doubting, the vision I had. Not one child, but two. It seemed as though things we should agree on to move forward became difficult in the beginning. Was she fully on board with the idea of having another child?

We knew we were both stronger because of what we had already endured. We would declare, "Yes, let's go ahead," and a few days later, we were not so sure.

At first, Nataliya and I were not in agreement about the transfer. Should we transfer one or both? This took a little time to work through. Knowledge, we needed knowledge, or we'd perish. I thought, *Why not both? Why only one if we're really going to do this?* I mean, last time we transferred two, and the result was one child. The reality of it all was before us once again. The myriad of questions rested on the limitation of choice. To not get lost or perish in the midst of making that choice. This would be our tour de force one more time.

There was a great deal of tension in making the choice. There were multiple possibilities for the outcome; there were only two embryos. The path was beckoning. Is this so difficult? The prospects would be none, one, or twins—a very real possibility if we transferred both.

Once again, we sought counsel about what to do and how to do it, based, this time, on the vast knowledge we had garnered. We chose Barbra again to be that neutral person, giving assistance not aligned with or supporting any side or position—an arbitrator, if you will. She listened to the apprehension we both had. Nataliya's fear was about the future trouble if we transferred both embryos. And my desires were about wanting to duplicate the result by following the path we went down before.

Steps of faith. Trusting God as we go. Details of the one-step, two-step progression. Stepping into the IVF ring again—the world of possibilities. Gestating hope during the weeks prior. Wandering while wondering if our hearts can make the journey again.

Prolific

The thoughts of increase (our quiver) caused a familiar trend for us. We found ourselves needing another bedroom on the main floor.

Abby would have a sister or brother to grow up with. Not just in thought alone, as it usually begins when making these kinds of decisions, but with a real increase to the family, the outcome of such decisions if they go this way, and the certain trials to meet along the way. Those faith variables, the increase of our progeny, with one that's not here yet, but thought about as if they were. Moving once again, stepping out in faith, our hearts now set on a quiver's fulfillment and a move to accommodate such—we're ready.

We did as before; we made plans to move, with the hope our family would grow once again. This time, however, we started building a new home without having to move first. No temporary apartment would be needed.

We would be living in our larger home prior to transferring the embryos. Faith needing faith—that first step.

Our plan was to list our current home about three months before the new home was due to be completed. Hoping for a fast sale, favor was on our side. The home sold quickly.

Once we moved into our new home, our plans of increase could move forward—two rooms on the main floor occupied, and a third holding a crib-in-waiting, and the rest that would be needed —all waiting.

After a few months, we were ready. We contacted our doctors again, the first step in the family-increase procession. Hoping. Knowing the direction we were going, the road lay before us, potholes and all, our feet to be planted upon it.

Together in alignment, once again on the same page, we decided to transfer two embryos, the only two we had left.

I, then fifty-six years old, and my wife, forty-three, were both on a beeline to get this process started, knowing how long it took before. Time rambles on, with no respect for people and not on our side. Our reflections in the mirror reminding us of time's assault.

Our hopes were high. Because we both believed that, by being good stewards with what the Lord had given us for future use, we should produce favor in the direction we were going with little trauma. Placing the responsibility alone on the Lord to provide.

Neglecting, I think, that life, as precious as it is, if things are not right genetically or within the womb and more, God might just say, "No, not yet." Another hidden grace that some just can't bear, but one that God allows. Truthfully, one rarely understood,

I think, that life sometimes just can't move forward, regardless of one's pursuit.

It leaves one to question, "Why no child yet?" Or the possibility that lingers. One of never-to-be as time flees in the face of wasted pursuit. Thoughts teeming. Tears welling. Sometimes the mind just can't digest what it's being fed. It is a difficult thing to learn about God's grace. Learning the outcome, and yet, sufficient in every way, because He knows the end prior to all beginnings, to get on board with that or stay on the sidelines. Of what He would save an individual from—grace—knowing very well what one can and some cannot abide.

Somehow this thought didn't compute in my "God's got this" scenario. The one I thought I was abiding in, I mean, because we're being good stewards. Or as I thought then, His favor should be ours. Talk about missing the mark. Man assuming what God will or will not do according to man's choice or timing—foolishness!

But as of then, we didn't know how things were going to work out for us. His favor being applied in so many ways we didn't even know. Ways, where if gain be not arrived to, and grace still win the day,God protection over us, covering both defeat and victory with a balm that heals.

A hard lesson? No one thinks this way, or at least I didn't. Again, a huge step of faith before us. Not just building a home for a future investment, but to have three rooms on the main floor for the more profound investment. One of posterity. A quiver becoming full.

Just so you know, for us, this was an all-or-nothing scenario. Transferring both embryos. If we became pregnant, then it would seem that all of our effort would be rewarded. If not, then we'd at least managed our responsibility, stewarding those embryos we had in our care. Discerning that, if no life comes through all the effort put forth—knowing very well the emotions that would be unhinged and the tears that must fall and would—the heartache of loss would be on full display once again. The Lord ministering to us and tending to our tears afterwards. We knew that He would apply grace (a balm) where it was most needed, our hearts. He would for some time care for what needed mending.

This theory of ours, stewardship equaling favor—I don't think the latter even computed. I mean, we never thought that we wouldn't get pregnant—just a gut feeling, I guess.

This is far different than the first part of this story. Where life is walking before us at two years old—our precious daughter in our midst. We never forget the path we took so that she might be here. The emotion I feel writing now is different than before; I know now exactly what the outcome is prior to writing about it. Unlike before, when I had no idea and was only presenting it in real time as it was unfolding one week to the next as you read. Our hearts on our sleeve, naked and exposed to outcome. And the human despair that accompanies such. Those who would pursue that path again—unknown courage.

Onward to Transfer

"There is some scar tissue on her uterus from the past pregnancy," they said. And so, like our preceding story, Nataliya would have to go in for surgery again.

The cost of stepping down this IVF road once more would be stifling at times, and not just financially. We were accompanied by doctors, nurses, and others who knew of our previous battle.

And yet, we stepped again, all of us, into the unknown, adhering to our faith to get us from one side to the other. We chose to trust that life would come forth.

Nataliya has been following some couples online, "observing them" in their IVF journey. I follow their stories from time to time, and more often than not, the stories I am drawn to and remember are the stories of great sadness. The failure stories. Maybe because those seem to be more prevalent than the successes you hear about. And likely, because of what we had been through before, wanting to see how others navigate through their trauma and loss. It is heartbreaking to watch people's online despair. More so because some are still trying after two, three, or more transfers.

This was our story, wearing the loss on our sleeves because our faces could not hide the disappointments, setbacks, and heartbreak. Maybe it is your story too—a story filled with many setbacks plaguing the journey.

The IVF journey unites those of us who choose to travel down that path—those in the online stories and those of you reading this book. We all want to bring a child into our lives.

IVF united us as we endured great loss, suffering together, remembering ours, and writing the events post-trauma. When failure pervades, penetrating all the way to the bone—theirs and ours—through trial we become united. The experience brings people closer together, while at the same time, they remain unknown to each other. Yet trauma, when such great defeat be upon people's hidden hopes, can sadly drive us apart at times.

Together

We keep stepping down the path, as do some of the online families we follow. We continue down the same path to the unknown, where life possibly waits.

Will life come forth or not? These are the questions that one continues to combat, reflecting an internal passion, our deepest hope—the IVF success story that everyone wants.

For us, for them, we trust that life will come forth, fulfilling a quiver's desire. For are we not known about, before we're even born, in the heart of God? We most certainly are. My wife and I are believers in the Lord Jesus. He plays a most significant role in our lives, and therefore our IVF journey. He knows perfectly well the outcome. He knows exactly where we are—this one-step, two-step progression, the march of faith. Growing two together through such trials. He is fully aware that one's passion for such ends up in one of two outcomes.

So now, Nataliya healed from the last surgery, my wife and I have a date with the embryologist for transferring the embryos. So strange, the thought of thawing embryos for transfer. One we've not yet encountered. A thought that most people will never consider in their lifetimes, except the few called to walk on this lonely road. It is right that the embryos are thought about, and carefully, at every step. As every placement of one's foot on this path, this IVF journey, it is a campaign that holds life in the balance as these little lives wait to make their entrance.

An acumination, a steadied course focused, walking by faith down to the sharpest thought—the quantum dimension where life hides and waits.

Will the embryo survive the trauma of thawing? Will it survive transfer? Life is so delicate and the entire process such a mystery. Will life come forth?

B-Day
(Baby Day)

Here we are, ready or not. The day of transfer has arrived! We are excited as we make our way into the same procedure room as before. The same brightly lit room, once again waiting, hoping, and praying the same as last time. That pins-and-needles interval, then ten days from now, we'll know. Life or not life?

Waiting and wondering, asking ourselves, *Will it be the same as last time?* There's no escaping it, these kinds of thoughts. Waiting… one day, two days, a few days more. My wife already making the important trip to the store, retrieving those home pregnancy tests. Testing on day four, five, and six with great anticipation. Each test telling a story of what might come. Shaking off the negative defeat, waiting for tomorrow to take another, hoping for the digital readout to be different than the day before.

Incredible! Incredible that life shows up in a test where the HCG hormone allows one to see if they are pregnant before the blood test at day nine.

A hope fulfilled with great joy hangs in the balance on that day. Yes, we found ourselves to be pregnant *that day*.

We lived in that joy for six glorious weeks until great sadness pervaded. Invading our hearts, befalling our hope—the balm needing to be applied once again. Life was no more in the womb where it had lain days before. Our hearts, broken.

Tears fell for weeks on end, it seemed. Groans that only God knows the meaning of. Our heads finding no rest on our pillows. No peace to be found in those first few days. Only the seat of emotion resting, grinding in the pit of our bellies. The gut-wrenching turmoil pervaded and would not stop. Life was no more.

> *Just as you'll never understand the mystery of life forming in a pregnant woman, So you'll never understand the mystery at work in all that God does. (Ecclesiastes 11:5)*

Our story, difficult as it was, is a story that is shared by many who are found on this path. This journey of hope. One into the quantum abyss, searching for life. Not knowing, and at the same time, the hope of adding a first child and for some, adding to a family not yet complete, as was ours. In the heart of those who long for more, a quiver not quite full yet, leaving questions of "what if?" That damned what-if!

Of course, at the onset of such loss, all that we could think about, even the next day—the same for most people I would suspect—was, *How?* How can we put life back where it lay the day before? Weeping. We just want what we had the day before. We want it now!

I was angry. I felt empty. We both did. Broken all over again, the same as before. We gave those babies names too. Never getting to meet them or hold them, love on them. The extra room, the crib, both lay vacant. Waiting for our hope to come forth, the silent tears pouring down our faces. Utter despair, bone-deep, the loss of another child.

For my wife, there were just no words to attend the great sadness she felt. During the first few days that followed, she withheld much. As I, too, would not share my grief fully yet, wanting to tear my clothes and throw ashes on my head. As if to hold on to it would change what's happened. It would not. I'm sure Nataliya felt as I did. Wanting life, and wanting it where it lay just days before, we were unable to shake that feeling.

The stories of so many on this journey, once again, are not all stories of great joy. For sadness is also a very present reality for many as we are submerged into that great sadness of loss more than once. Not that there wasn't success for us, for Abby did come into our lives at our second attempt during round two of our first IVF venture. Noting again round one, still remembering the pain of loss at a balloon ceremony, and round three, our second IVF journey, trying to succeed afterwards in the midst of loss.

Yet revisiting that pain when looking at an empty room and crib, as it was upon us again. Just no words, sitting in an empty room with an empty crib, weeping. But knowing there was hope was difficult to ascertain. Needing to believe. Not an empty hope, but a certain hope was out there. A hope that God has grown us through thus far. Nothing wasted. He has shown us more and more how precious life really is.

For us, even from the point of transfer, all three times, we'd already picked out names, calling forth life before a breath was even taken. From the deepest parts of our souls, we did this. The hidden place, then into the womb, still calling by name, heralding that child come forth. We hoped as many do, and probably always will—we called them by name.

One element of this calling forth by name when praying for this little soul was a hope that her life would be added to our quiver afterwards. Violated—at least, that is how I felt when life was no more in that safe place, the womb. And the pain, never more real, left scars on our souls. *The sadness, no greater thing to know than this kind of loss.* A great difficulty reserved for those who would step onto the path of IVF.

Real Time–Once Again

So here we are again, trying to put life back where life once lay. No longer trying to fix what couldn't be fixed, mind you. But yes, stepping once again onto the path where life can be found. Through the grace of God, we are given another chance for life to come forth. He has given us the means and fortitude to make the venture one more time. The great undertaking—to pursue life, calling by name, knowing we may, or may not, find what we're looking for, but we take the chance anyway.

Some might ask, "Is it worth the pain to go through another round of IVF, knowing the possibilities?" And with an obvious fear, having experienced both sides now, the outcome on both fronts, to trust to endeavor once more?

Well, for us, still feeling that our family was not yet complete, yes, it's worth it. For us to try one more time, knowing that this could turn into two, or maybe even three more attempts, due to the number of embryos we might have if success is not found in the beginning.

The bigger question to be asked is, "Where does one stop?" Hoping to have another child, to be successful, we would continue moving forward until we just couldn't move anymore.

However, at this time, I don't believe that either of us is compelled to make a demand of the other. We feel our role is to steward and to do so carefully until they're all gone, even if we end up with more than needed.

No, I believe the Lord has a different plan this time if there are remaining embryos. A plan that He'll make clear as time goes on. He will make it known to us what must be done.

Made Known

Therefore, with this newfound drive to move forward in the face of trauma, through the loss occurring the last time, we are now ready to step onto the path again. Not only are we ready, but today, December 1, 2019, our hope is that, well, maybe we can be pregnant by February 2020, and birth by Abby's fourth birthday. That way, she might have a little sister or brother to grow up with, our quiver will increase and be full with the vision we've been given. Hope! We have hope.

• • •

Today is February 11, 2020, and we're not there yet, but we are on our way. We have made it through another harvest and have fertilized, having more than we did the first two times. Amazing!

The further down this path that God has taken us, the more we are learning to trust Him in ways we never could or would before. The world we live in has changed. We're learning how to cope and live with a pandemic! COVID-19 has come onto the world scene during our pursuit of life.

How will this impact our journey? We do not know yet. Since February, however, the impact of COVID-19 on the world has become something no one thought could ever be. We may have to put the brakes on.

We have just been told that elective surgeries are going to be put on hold starting in mid-March, and if we are going to transfer, that we need to make up our minds right now, or the window will be closed, not knowing when it will open again for elective surgeries, which IVF is.

So we've made a choice. A choice made in the midst of a pre-COVID-19 world, as this is the way we are going—we have chosen life in the midst of such ubiquitous turbulence. To pursue life—and that it would come forth even during a world's parturition, birth pains, and the delivery and propagation found in the 2020 COVID-19 world pandemic. A worldwide birth of great tribulation, and life's finding its way through, while at the same time, many lives are being lost to the pandemic.

Life

Two days ago, Tuesday, March 17, 2020, we transferred one of the embryos, and now we wait. But not in fear, even with all that's going on in the world right now. We are, by grace, seemingly steadied. We are excitedly blessed with another chance of life coming forth into our hearts and home. A home that has been waiting for another little life to occupy it. One to complete our hopes.

• • •

It became apparent soon after the transfer that life was not meant to be at this time. We have been here before, and it is no less heartbreaking this time.

With the shutdown of elective procedures, we are left wondering when we may have another chance.

The entire world is in the middle of a pandemic that has taken thousands of lives already. Could it get any worse with one more? We don't even know what could've happened if we became pregnant in the beginnings of this. Could it have been worse, contracting coronavirus, and how might that affect a baby in the womb? No one really knows the full extent of what could happen.

It's been a dreadful virus thus far. One that has killed over nine hundred thousand people in America alone at this time and over six million worldwide, thousands more dying every day. When will it stop?

Maybe that was God's grace. Providing naught for us in the womb this time may have been a blessing; only God knows. We usually don't think about His blessing that way—not getting what we want being a good thing.

Stepping onto that lonely road again, the uncertainty prevailing, it is a very present feeling. That road into the quantum realm—one of not seeing, not hearing, and not knowing—but stepping onto it anyway, the outcome strangely anonymous. Faith, a step forward carefully, hoping not to trip. What really happens in this place of why or why not—the darkness called quantum where life—and, further, that first breath—waits?

We know only one thing for sure—that we're both ready to transfer another embryo as soon as we can. And at the same time, not knowing when that time will come, the quantum reach deepens within both of us, beckoning life, asking that same question again found in the beginning of these writings—when?

•••

The pandemic is in full swing now, and with all that's happening, possibility is delayed as we must wait a little longer. What will happen next? Will we become pregnant? We don't know. We do know that we hope, the same hope we always had along this journey. And coronavirus or not, we truly believe that we'll become parents again to another precious little one in the midst of such, as soon as elective surgeries are allowed again.

July 2020
Our Journey Continues

Four months have passed, and it's now the beginning of July. We received a phone call from our doctor, who said, "Elective surgeries are now being allowed again." So excited to hear the news that we scheduled our appointment date.

On that day, we transferred one of the remaining embryos we had left. And, of course, there was another wait in the grand scheme of our desire, believing it to be God's desire and His best for us. Still asking, Will life come forth this time? Contemplating it not only could, but would, and in the depth of a worldwide pandemic.

• • •

Yes!

We are found to be with child again! Grateful be the song in our hearts. And our prayers answered. We are pregnant! Hallelujah!

To say those words, "We are pregnant," and in the midst of a pandemic, one that has tattered the lives of so many others. Taking pieces of life and life itself; shattering people's dreams, hopes, plans, jobs. Permanently changing their course, their families. But our course, too, has changed. Even in the midst of this chaos, there was a certain calm that only God could give.

So here we are; in the next two weeks, we go for a sonogram to hear our baby's heartbeat for the first time. It seems for me that, biologically, I am more prone to produce females since my other biological children are female.

We call out her name before we truly know her. Her name is Ella! Doing just like we have before. With just a few cells, we not only saw them at her genesis, but we did the same once more, choosing between them, which cells (embryo) prior to transferring—a view into this hidden reach where life abides. The quantum realm, life coming forth, responding softly with a heart-beat as if to say, "I'm here." The genesis of life, truly a gift, this choosing, we are so humbled. Several embryos this time, the Lord was saying to us, "You choose." We did, knowing my predisposition, my proclivity to produce females—not fully knowing that we'd chosen Ella at that time. Her name not known until after the transfer.

Chapter 28

Taken by Faith

For those of you who are on the same journey we've been on, we pray for your success. We know very well that the road before you is not an easy one. A road well-worn with much pacing and fretting. A road that has become very narrow for others. One where you might feel as if you're walking uphill through wet concrete. Struggling to continue after so much presumed failure, as we were subjected to. But we also discovered that, when navigating the uncertainty of IVF, endeavoring one's heart to this course, tears must fall in joy and in sorrow. And you, too, will discover this while pursuing life with the possibility of not-life at the same time. A most travailing impact on one's heart. Such is life—to live knowing one day that the end will come. One that awaits those who will endeavor IVF, undertaking that venture. And yes, to all of us who live the multiplicity of engagements. Truly a gift, even with that end in view—the end of life. The outcome teaches one to grow in ways that they never would. And for those who will, to trust in God in ways they never could have before. Calling out His name to both fronts.

For the few who are called to this path, the road to in vitro fertilization, a bravery becomes born in one's soul. What is brought forth is something that was not there before. It is the possibility of life, and in demanding that life, steps of courage must be taken to procure it. Taken by faith. Secured with a future hope always in mind that life will prevail. And the irony found in seeking life through this process is that there will be steps that are not yet known to the one who steps this way. Going places they never would have gone before—IVF leading.

Chapter 29

Second Trimester

We are now four months along, walking down the path that IVF patrons follow. Through, over, under, and around. Doing our best. Planning for what God has put His hand to, leading us, and without knowing at times that we are even being led. Today is my fifty-eighth birthday. I am writing with great joy as we've entered our second trimester. I am blessed and happy because Nataliya is beginning to feel a bit better. Her body no longer drenched with the influx of hormones—progesterone, estrogen patches, etc. There are fewer bad days now and more good ones.

Our last sonogram went well. All the measurements taken, they told us everything was normal. Thankful.

Praying for Ella with our three-and-a-half-year-old daughter—this, too, a joy untold. Where thoughts uttered, hearing Abby call her name aloud, "Ella, Ella!" What joy we are having, sharing Ella with Abby before Ella's arrival. Telling Abby that Ella is inside mommy's tummy, growing, that she'll be here in another five months to meet her. She smiles, not really understanding, but knows we are happy as she joins in, calling her name— "Ella, Ella!"

Chapter 30

Joy

We do not observe these moments passively. Especially knowing that we are experiencing something, percentagewise, that few have experienced. The first IVF baby, Louise Brown, was born on July 25, 1978, at Oldham General Hospital in the United Kingdom. The first "test-tube baby," they called her. A term depictive of the process, but it lost its scientific epithet later. It was life, human life!

IVF now allows life to come forth for those who in no other way could become parents. Egg and seed merge, becoming the dictionary definition of vitality: "Capacity for survival or for the continuation of a meaningful or purposeful existence, the power to live and grow." Therefore, yielding offspring outside of adoption is now made possible for those who could not have their own children otherwise. For many, the egg and sperm generated from their own stock, prior to 1978, was just a thought speculative of possibility, not yet a reality.

Since then, at the time of this writing, just eight million[7] plus children have come into the world through IVF.

With seven and a half billion people on the planet, those who go through IVF successfully are a very small percentage of the gross population. Not that one child is more valuable than the next, once in the womb, but for those parents who have had to endure this journey, I believe special attention is given afterwards, remembering how they arrived here. One that is natural to few, again, respectively to the gross population.

God has indeed set the stage for something very special—the IVF journey. "To be fruitful and multiply," God proclaimed over humanity and allowed new ways to help make that happen. A place where hope is found once again, seeded by God. The great conceptive possibility—IVF.

Almost no one chooses the IVF path first. Instead, it is chosen when all hope has been dashed against the rocky crags, despairing one's hopes, year after year, regarding the natural order of gestating, and not just the idea of childbirth. The way the world generally conceives is accidental so many times, not planned, and then the child is actually carried, from beginning to end, and delivered, not discarded—hence, a natural order. Having that order of things come true for those found on this IVF path is an astonishing journey, to say the least. And the value placed upon such is utterly profound, as I've experienced.

Yes, God's hand is in it all the way. Whether one believes it or not, believes in God or not, it is with great hope and grit

---

[7] https://www.sciencedaily.com/releases/2018/07/180703084127.htm

that a heart sustains this journey for many. Even softened along the way, as this would be my hope when they find life thriving through this unnatural order, as we did—the IVF journey. God made a way where there was no way for us. I hope that those on this journey discover this truth—a valuable truth in more ways than truly known.

Chapter 31

A Journey Filled with Every Emotion

Moving onward through the first trimester and the stage-setting elements, those that squeeze one's sanity emerge! They do calm down afterwards for most IVF patrons. Having no more progesterone shots and estrogen patches. Those essentials necessary to the process that exhaust and fatigue, debilitating one's sanity at times. Then the second trimester, becoming what most tend to think of as normal—an ordinary pregnancy. Regardless, normal, if such a thing exists through this process.

In the beginning, as abnormal does, it beckons a remembrance, as most will never forget how the journey began for them, the how to get this process started. More so for those who were unsuccessful and never forgot the downside. To not try again after one, two, and for some, three or more heart-wrenching attempts is the beginning of lost hope. One they suffer with PTSD. This was our experience, and more, through the multiple harvest of eggs and transfers that failed, a journey filled with every emotion, severe anxiety, pain, and joy. All swirling around at the same time in a sea of quantum influx. Flowing in and out, systematic emotions throughout an ordered cause and effect.

• • •

We've just passed the four-month mark—seventeen weeks and five days, to be exact. The time going much quicker now.

• • •

Continuing in hope, faithfully strengthened to the call upon us, as this coming Monday will be nineteen weeks and four days—the halfway mark. We are scheduled to see the doctor for exact measurements of the baby's size—and to discover the sex as well.

• • •

The results of our visit—we couldn't be happier. The measurements were in the normal range. Such a sigh of relief combed over us. Certainly, and natural for many, those inward confidential speculating inquiries. Those that plague prior to this day. Wondering, Will everything be okay—the appointments' conclusions? What if they aren't? I suspect that it's natural for many to think this way. And more so, especially for those who are our age.

Then the results. The baby weighs eleven ounces, and the heartbeat is 154 beats per minute. "Very normal," the doctor said as relief calmed our journey's fare. The turbulence finally coming to rest.

• • •

Perfect. Everything was perfect. We've just passed the twenty-one-week mark. Continuing in the faith given to us, we are thankful with all that we are.

The doctor's reports continue with confidence that all is well and normal.

Chapter 32

The Third *T*

We now find ourselves in the beginning of the third trimester. 28 weeks and on the cusp of Christmas week. The third "t" signifying "trimester," and having a deeper semblance hidden at the arrival too, this third trimester and the conclusion thereafter. Thankfulness being multiplied, the emotion that reigns in both our lives at this time. How far we've come.

Setting our course in the beginning, one child was all that was in our hearts and on our minds. Two years and eleven months to get there, and now, a second child almost here, two years and three months from our first thought to do this one more time. Yes, we set our course. A course that most certainly changed along the way. Obvious now to both of us, the contents of one's heart. Do we truly know what's hidden in there? I think deep down only the Lord knows what's hidden in the depths of our hearts. We can both see that we have been led through this entire journey. Upon catastrophic failure at times, about what to do next, and then doing it, not knowing what outcome awaited. We now know those options were all provided by the One who was leading us. The One who set this whole thing up from the beginning, at an MPC conference back in January 2014.

Chapter 33

One Week
or Less

Dilated to one centimeter, we wait for our next appointment five days from now.

•••

Having left that appointment, we are still one centimeter. Today is Tuesday, and next Tuesday evening we are scheduled to go into the hospital if we make it that long without going into labor. Two days before the forty-week mark. There is a strange calm throughout our home, awaiting Ella's arrival. One week from now, or sooner, she will come into our lives. The struggle is coming to an end. Grateful is the reigning thought. Thinking about loving another person coming into our home. Our four-year-old having been that person and the center of attention with all our affection to date. As time draws near, however, both of us now excited to hold and love Ella. She too will be the center of our attention and with all our affection, as there is enough to go around.

The promises of God are so much more than we could ever know, as implied earlier in the writing. His question in the beginning to my wife Nataliya, "Who made the choice when you said you were done having children? Was that Me—God—or you who made that choice without Me?" Our narrow vision circumscribed at the beginning of all of this. Our understanding singular. All we could think about was one child being added to our family, not seeing more. We realized later, after Abby was born, that when God spoke to my wife, He specifically used the word "children," the plural of "child," and our hearts moved, accomplishing what He spoke over us. Not one child but two fulfilling the vision I had, walking down the hall at our apartment, even before the first child arrived. I was in the middle, holding the hand of a child on my left and a child on my right.

Bless the name of God! His vision always greater than what we see for ourselves. Bless the name of God! His provision more abundant, more fruitful, more in every way. From no way possible, as was our IVF beginning, to then quantum leap, transilience, and ultimate boundaries that confined us, pierced our hearts, arriving at the truth of God's vision for us—not one, but two, our quiver now forever full.

Chapter 34

Arrived

She's here!

We went into the hospital Tuesday evening at 6:30, and on Wednesday morning, 11:49, Ella was born. So incredible to be witness to such a miracle. I've never seen or been part of something so breathtaking. Intense joy upon delivery. The first breath of air that follows—nothing on earth compares.

Chapter 35

A Message of Hope

There is nothing about our story that others on the IVF path have not encountered. Many will never write about it though. It's because of the privacy that seems to go hand in hand with IVF, unlike the natural way, with little or no trauma shared before all. But IVF, the difficulties, the loss at times, the intense emotion that tends to follow through the process—maybe it's too painful to remember all they went through, arriving at where they are now. Gain or loss, privacy seems to beckon for many. Maybe it's something else.

Regardless, I have written this story to encourage others on the IVF path, to say that there is *hope*! Our story, as painful as it was, has had many mountaintop moments. To plow through, to keep going, to use all the resources that are available. To hope! To further hope! Grateful for all of it!

Medicine and IVF techniques are evolving and improving every day. Some of the procedures we encountered may not be your experience, or even used any more. I'm sure there are many new theories and methods being introduced, even at this writing. This book is not meant as an education on the medical techniques. It is written in the hopes that our story will give you comfort along your journey. And although every journey is different, you do not have to travel the path alone.

Skilled professionals can prepare you for what to expect in the process, but they do not prepare you for the emotional and spiritual journey you will take. Faith is the secret ingredient they do not share with you. Faith will be your strength. He will be your rod and your staff. He has brought you to this point, and He will see you through it.

> *Don't you see that children are God's best gift? The fruit of the womb his generous legacy? (Psalms 127:3)*

www.ingramcontent.com/pod-product-compliance
Lightning Source LLC
Chambersburg PA
CBHW072233290326
41934CB00008BA/1276